ABOUT THE BOOK AND THE AUTHORS

Petr Skrabanek was born in Bohemia where he studied natural sciences and later worked as a forensic toxicologist, while James McCormick spent twenty years in general practice. Petr's education was in communist schools, while James was educated in the liberal ambience of Cambridge. The vicissitudes of life made Petr complete medical studies in Ireland and spend a few years in clinical medicine before getting involved in endocrine oncology research and neuro-transmitters. James had meanwhile been translated from a rural practice to academia as head of a University Department of Community Health. While Petr has kept irritating medical authorities, James has become one, first Dean of the School of Physic in Trinity College (his authority further strengthened by the quaintness of the title) and more recently President of the Irish College of General Practitioners.

Petr teaches a course on critical appraisal of medical evidence in James's department, while James is free to pursue his interests in epidemiology, medical sociology, health services, and medical education. To escape from reality, Petr runs a postgraduate course on 'Finnegans Wake' in the Department of English of the rival University in Dublin, while James, to be in touch with reality, still cares for a small number of patients.

The authors say of *Follies and Fallacies in Medicine* :

'The aim of our book is to reach inquisitive minds, particularly those who are still young and uncorrupted by dogma. We offer no solutions to the problems we raise because we do not pretend to know of any. Both of us have been thought to suffer from scepticaemia* but are happy to regard this affliction, paradoxically, as a health promoting state. Should we succeed in infecting others we will be well content'.

*Scepticaemia: An uncommon generalised disorder of low infectivity. Medical school education is likely to confer life-long immunity.

FOLLIES AND FALLACIES IN MEDICINE

Petr Skrabanek
James McCormick

THE TARRAGON PRESS
Glasgow

ISBN 1 870781 02 3

A CIP catalogue record for this book is available from the British Library.

Cover design by Janet Hewitt

Typeset in 10pt Palatino by Tarragon Press
Printed by Gilmour and Lawrence, Glasgow

TABLE OF CONTENTS

TABLE OF CONTENTS   i

ACKNOWLEDGEMENTS   vi

INTRODUCTION   1

CHAPTER 1: PLACEBOS   3

Introduction   3

The placebo effect   4

Disease and illness   6

Asher's Paradox   7

Secrecy surrounding placebos   8

Placebo experiments   10

Quantifying the placebo effect   10

The milieu and the placebo, and the Clever Hans

phenomenon   14

The placebo effects of therapeutically active drugs   16

The assessment of drugs   17

Pain and the placebo response   18

Conclusion   20

CHAPTER 2 : A FISTFUL OF FALLACIES 21

Introduction 21

The fallacy of association being causal 21

The ecological fallacy 26

Surrogate-outcome fallacy 28

The faggot fallacy 30

The weight-of-evidence fallacy 30

The Bellman's fallacy 32

The fallacy of authority 32

The fallacy of 'everybody says so' 36

The fallacy of simple explanation 37

The magic bullet fallacy 38

The bad-blood fallacy 39

The fallacy of risk 40

The fallacy of inappropriate extrapolation 42

The fallacy of the golden mean 43

Fallacies in randomised controlled studies 43

The Beethoven fallacy 45

The new syndrome fallacy 46

The fallacy of insignificant significance 47

The fallacy of post-hoc statistics 48

The fallacy of 'positive' results 49

Error of the third degree 50

The fallacy of obfuscation 51

The fallacy of covert bias 53

The 'Gold Effect' fallacy 54

The 'hush, hush' fallacy 56

The fallacy of experience 57

CHAPTER 3 : DIAGNOSIS AND LABELLING 59

Introduction 59

The diagnostic process 60

The need for diagnosis 61

Benefits of diagnosis 62

Sick role 62

Diagnostic error 63

Levels of diagnosis 64

Diagnosis in psychological and social terms 64

Physical disease 65

Non-disease 66

Koro 70

Obesity 70

Hypertension 72

Harms of labelling 74

Psychiatric disease 75

Psychiatric diagnosis 77

A lunacy of labels 78

The surgery of labels 82

The translation game 84

Conclusion 85

CHAPTER 4 : PREVENTION   87

The fallacy that prevention is always better than
cure   87

The fallacy of cheating death   88

Limits imposed by ignorance   90

The fallacy of multifactorial aetiology   90

Successful prevention   92

Coronary heart disease   93

The evidence that altering 'risk factors'
diminishes coronary heart disease   95

Screening for cancer   99

Screening for breast cancer   100

Screening for cancer of the uterine cervix   103

The abominable no-men   106

Prevention parodies   107

Prevention as a crusade   108

The ethical dimension   109

CHAPTER 5 : ALTERNATIVE MEDICINE   113

The nature of alternative therapies   114

Homoeopathy   115

Bach's flower remedies   119

Acupuncture   120

Electroquackupuncture devices   122

Osteopathy and chiropractic   123

Miraculous healing   125

Christian Science   128

Psychic surgery   130

Radiesthesia, radionics, psionic medicine   132

Conclusion   134

CHAPTER 6 : MORALITY AND MEDICINE   135

Medicine and science   135

The moral dimension   137

Morality and the public health   139

CHAPTER 7 : ENVOI   143

REFERENCES :   147

Chapter 1   147

Chapter 2   150

Chapter 3   155

Chapter 4   159

Chapter 5   162

Chapter 6   168

Chapter 7   169

ACKNOWLEDGEMENTS

Books do not arise of themselves; they do not emerge from the primeval slime but are grafted on to some bizarre selection of everything that has gone before, a selection which is determined by the past experience of their authors. It follows that we are only able to acknowledge a few of the many who are responsible for what has been written and eventually printed.

A number of friends and colleagues have been kind enough to read earlier drafts and to criticise and encourage in varying proportions: they include Shane Allwright, Iain Chalmers, Thomas Sherwood, William Silverman and our wives. We are also grateful to Diane Hughes and to her anonymous reviewers whose criticism has been invaluable.

Finally, we are grateful to David Sumner who provided encouragement, criticism and was a most sympathetic and enthusiastic publisher, to Joyce Bermingham for her patience with innumerable drafts and demands, and to the WR Nunn Memorial Trust for support.

INTRODUCTION

'The chief cause of poverty in science is imaginary wealth. The chief aim of science is not to open a door to infinite wisdom but to set a limit to infinite error'.

Bertolt Brecht, *Galileo*.

This book is about setting a limit to medical error. Not the kind of error which leads to the amputation of the wrong limb or which leads to the 'dead' coming to life in the mortuary. Such error is human and inevitable. The kinds of error with which we are concerned are errors of doctrine, systematic errors which are part of dogma and accepted truth, distortions which set obstacles in the path of rational thought and enquiry. The progress of science and the growth of knowledge depend upon clearing away rubbish and challenging accepted dogma and belief. Although we run the risk of being labelled, in William Silverman's phrase, as 'nihilists intent on subverting medicine's high purpose', our purpose is not to criticise medicine or those who practice it, but to advocate the need for criticism *in* medicine. Doctors, aided by scientists, can, by honest admission of ignorance, by demystifying rituals and by rational inquiry, discover new ways and improve old ways of easing our journey from the cradle to the grave.

Chapter one hauls the placebo from the medical cupboard and shows that it is still much more than a skeleton. Chapter two is a mini-zoo of treacherous creepy-crawlies which interfere with the logical circuits in our brains. Chapter three examines the nature of diagnosis and the results of attaching labels. Chapter four is concerned with present enthusiasm for prevention, its limits and possibilities. Chapter five acupunctures, painlessly we hope, the blisters of 'alternative' solutions which are disfiguring the face of rational medicine. Chapter six touches on ethical issues and the boundaries between morality and medicine. Chapter seven offers a brief envoi, designed to restore some measure of content to the disturbed.

This book derives, at least in part, from our teaching responsibilities, which include introducing students to critical appraisal. A small group format encourages open, friendly and intimate discussion, which is suitable for exploring subjects that are often neglected in the ordinary course of medical teaching: such things as the nature of medical evidence, deception in medical practice, money and medicine, ethics, and medicine as an institution of social control. We have learned at least as much as our students from this experience and have often joined each other in class in order to criticise each other's prejudices.

Our intent has been to provide an accessible book rather than a technical treatise and it is certainly not meant to be a text-book. Our goal is a plain man's guide to the limitations of medicine.

1

PLACEBOS

Introduction

The *Bristol Journal* of December 23rd 1988 reports that a new clinic has been established which claims to boost people's energy and restore virility with injections of pig embryos and horses' blood. 'Harley Street specialist Peter Stephen charges an amazing £1,500 for a course of 'Swiss natural biological treatments' .....'.   Another news item reports that 'Dr Stephen drives a BMW and has recently purchased a large house in a fashionable neighbourhood'.

In the twenties, Professor Eugene Steinach of Vienna introduced vasectomy as a rejuvenating procedure, his rationale being that as loss of sperm had a debilitating effect (a popular belief), it would surely be the case that blockage of the loss would have invigorating results. As a result of the 'success' of this operation over one hundred teachers and university professors underwent the procedure. Their number included Sigmund Freud and the poet W. B. Yeats.

The history of medicine is full of similar and equally extraordinary examples, all of which are based on the fallacy that an alteration in symptoms following treatment is necessarily a specific result of that therapy.   Nonetheless such is the need of both patients and doctors to believe in treatment that this assumption is widespread and is a potent cause of delusion. This chapter explores the nature of this phenomenon and tries to explain why otherwise rational people are prepared to put their faith in injections of extracts of pig embryos.

The placebo effect

There are three possible explanations for an association between treatment and cure. The first is that the treatment has actually had a beneficial effect. The second is the healing power of nature, the self-limiting nature of many ills, and the spontaneous improvement or return to health which would have taken place in the absence of any intervention. This 'vis medicatrix naturae' has been a most faithful ally of the medical profession throughout all ages: an ally lacking any licence to practice but providing a most valuable second opinion when called upon. Since the patient is rarely introduced to this benefactor - an 'éminence grise' who is consulted in secret - doctors acquire credit for the extraordinary ability of the human organism to overcome infection and many other insults.

The third explanation for benefit following therapy is the placebo effect. The word placebo, literally 'I will please', has been defined as 'an inert substance given for its psychological effect to satisfy the patient'. This definition is not completely satisfactory because the placebo effect may be exercised by substances which are not inert, and the placebo effect can be exercised in ways which do not involve the giving of medicines.

The term placebo first appears in its medical sense in the 19th century, although the idea goes back to time immemorial. In an editorial 'The placebo in medicine' in the *Medical Press* in 1890, the editor refers to the case of a lady who disputed her practitioner's bill. He had charged her for morphine while he had injected water. The lady won a court action against the doctor. The editor comments: 'We feel sorry for it, but apparently the law does not think well of placebos, and if the law does not like these gentle but useful members of the pharmaceutical community, well, the fact must be admitted that the knell of the placebo has been sounded. But what great good have they not effected in their generation! Think of the mild, undemonstrative, nevertheless soul-stirring, 'pillula panis' (the bread pill rolled between the fingers and covered with sugar). Shall it never again come to the aid of the oppressed female hysteric - never again have an opportunity of exerting its wonderful psychological effects as faithfully as one of its more toxic congeners? Then again, there is our old friend, 'Aq. Menth. Pip', (that is, peppermint water). Of this it can only be said that the good it has done will live after it'.[1]

The physician's belief in his treatment and the patient's faith in his physician exert a mutually reinforcing effect; the result is a powerful remedy which is almost guaranteed to produce an improvement and sometimes a cure. As a rule, discussions of the placebo effect concentrate on the gullibility of patients but ignore the self-deception of physicians. Platt wryly observed that the frequency with which placebos were used varied inversely with the combined intelligence of the doctor and his patient.[2]

In most present day instances the placebo is an antibiotic, a tonic, a cough bottle, a tranquilliser or other psychotropic, or some other compound which has pharmacological effects but whose beneficial results are not related to its pharmacological properties. National Formularies and other aids to prescribing do not list any placebos as such so that doctors are reduced to prescribing active compounds, even though they may recognise that the indications are weak and that any good effects are likely to be mediated through the placebo effect. It has been estimated that 35 - 45% of modern day prescriptions are unlikely to have any specific effects on the diseases for which they are ordered.[3] Patients who receive treatment are readily persuaded that they are having appropriate therapy and doctors may be deluded into believing that their prescribing is having specific effects. This results in a 'folie à deux' afflicting patient and doctor alike. Another unfortunate consequence is that large amounts of public and private money are being wasted because pharmaceuticals are much more expensive than sugar pills.

Disease and illness

For many people disease and illness are almost synonyms. It is nonetheless useful to make a distinction between what people feel (illness) and the existence of a pathological process (disease). Disease may or may not be accompanied by illness. Many diseases, including some that are potentially serious, are often symptomless; on the other hand, feeling unwell is not always the result of disease. Placebos have no effect on the progress or outcome of disease but they may exert a powerful effect upon the subjective phenomena of illness, pain, discomfort and distress. Their success is based upon this fact.

Pills and potions are not a necessary condition of the placebo effect. K. B. Thomas, a Southampton general practitioner, investigated the value of placebo prescribing in 200 of his patients. He identified those patients who had symptoms, such as headache, vague abdominal pain, backache, sore throats, coughs and tiredness, but in whom he was unable to make a specific diagnosis.[4] He first of all created two groups: one group received a 'positive consultation', that is they were offered a firm 'diagnosis' and strong reassurance that they would speedily recover. The second group were told, 'I cannot be certain what is the matter with you, but if you are not better within a few days please return'. The groups were further sub-divided in that half of the patients in each group were given a prescription. At the end of two weeks, 64% of those who had received a positive consultation were better as compared with only 39% of those who were offered uncertainty. 53% of those who received treatment were better as compared with 50% of those who had not received a prescription. This illustrates that the effect of the doctor as a placebo may be more powerful than the placebo effect of medicines.

Asher's paradox

Richard Asher, a distinguished London physician who achieved fame through the elegance and wit of his writing, pointed out that the success of therapy depends as much on the enthusiasm of the therapist as upon the faith of the patient. He went on to say: 'If you can believe fervently in your treatment, even though controlled studies show that it is quite useless, then your results are much better, your patients are much better, and your income is much better too. I believe this accounts for the remarkable success of some of the less gifted, but more credulous members of our profession, and also for the violent dislike of statistics and controlled tests which fashionable and successful doctors are accustomed to display'. [5]

There is a wider corollary to this phenomenon. Kenneth Galbraith in his *Anatomy of Power* observed that 'power accrues not to the individual who knows; it goes to the one who, often out of obtuseness, believes that he knows and who can persuade others to that belief'.

A *Lancet* editorialist asked 'Why is it deceitful to give a placebo if a large element of modern therapeutics is no better than a placebo? Is the gullibility of a good-hearted doctor preferable to (and more ethical than) the scepticism of one whose prescription is pharmacologically inert, when the results are the same?' [6]

The question remains: if a therapy is beneficial to the patient why should it be abandoned because some scientists, envious of its excellent results, accuse the doctors of using a placebo? This is the core of Asher's paradox: 'It is better to believe in therapeutic nonsense than openly to admit therapeutic bankruptcy. Better in the sense that a little credulity makes us better doctors, though worse research workers .... if you admit to yourself that the treatment you are giving is frankly inactive, you will inspire little confidence in your patients, unless you happen to be a remarkably gifted actor, and the results of your treatment will be negligible'.[7]

Secrecy surrounding placebos
Since much of the success of medicine, and to some extent the success of surgery, depends upon the placebo effect, it is puzzling that medical textbooks have little or nothing to say on the subject. Perhaps as has been observed 'the giving of a placebo seems to be a function of the physician, which like certain other functions of the body, is not to be mentioned in polite society'.[8] Most probably it represents a reluctance within the profession to face an embarrassing reality.

Despite the veil of secrecy which surrounds the placebo effect, some laymen have always been sceptical about the claims of physicians. Montaigne had this to say: 'For what reason do doctors arouse the credulity of their patients with false promises of cure other than to make their fraudulent nostrums work through the effect of the imagination? They know that one of the masters of their trade has written that there are people for whom the mere sight of medicine effects a cure'.[9]

While we now know that the cures of Hippocrates were due to the natural healing power of the body, augmented by the placebo effect, rather than being due to specific remedies, even in the Hippocratic age there were doubters. They accused Hippocratic physicians of self-deception, pointing out that their patients died or were helped because of luck rather than as a consequence of the 'art of healing': not surprisingly such gadflies were dismissed by the authors of the Hippocratic corpus as either 'delirious' or 'mad'.[10] Theophrastus in his *Enquiry into Plants*, written in the 3rd century B.C., accused those healers who claimed that their plants had magical properties of trying to glorify their own craft by telling lies.[11]

The principles of treatment of many common diseases have not changed much since the time of Hippocrates. Take for example treatment of the 'flu'. In the old days the excessive humour, or the daemon of the disease, would be purged by evacuation, bloodletting, sweating, emetics or enemas. Nowadays, the germs are 'washed out': 'Go to bed and take plenty to drink'. Cecil Helman, surveying folk beliefs about colds, chills and fevers in a London suburb, showed how modern therapeutics reinforces primitive beliefs.[12] 'The flu' attacks the person when 'the germ' or 'the virus', which are used as synonyms, 'goes around'. The germ can move around from one part of the body to another; it may start as a sore throat and 'go down' to the chest or lodge in the muscles. If it is on the chest, the best way to get rid of it is to wash it out with a cough bottle. Six million gallons of cough mixtures are prescribed every year in Britain alone to do exactly that, to get the germ off the chest, to help people to cough up the muck that contains the germ. If the germ moves to the stomach, it grows to the size of a bug and the bug is flushed out with fluids. 'Sweating it out' is considered nowadays as folk medicine and most physicians would regard such a prescription as beneath them; nonetheless most doctors will advise keeping warm.

Placebo experiments

Blackwell and his colleagues described an experiment which they carried out with the help of a group of medical students. Fifty six students were given either a pink or a blue sugar pill and told that the pills were either sedative or stimulant. Only three of the fifty six reported that the pills had no effect. Most of those who received the blue pills thought that they were sedative and 72% felt drowsy. Furthermore those who took two pills felt more drowsy than those who had only taken one. On the other hand 32% of those students who had taken the pink placebo said that they felt 'less tired'. One third of the students reported side effects which ranged from headaches, dizziness and watery eyes to abdominal discomfort, tingling extremities and staggering gait.[13]

In another study medical students in Canada were asked to participate in testing a new drug. Although all students received nothing more than a sugar pill, three quarters of them reported side effects which included depression, sedation, restlessness, excitation, tremors, headache and slowing of the heart beat.[14] If this arouses anxiety about the ethics of such experiments, it should be pointed out that it was part of an educational exercise.

Addiction to placebos is not uncommon. Many people are convinced of the benefit which they derive from the daily addition of vitamins or other substances to their already adequate diets.

Quantifying the placebo effect

Sir Douglas Black, a past president of the Royal College of Physicians, estimated that only about 10% of diseases are significantly influenced by modern treatment.[15] This echoes the opinion of Sir George Pickering, who guessed that in some 90% of patients seen by a general practitioner the effects of treatment are unknown or there is no specific remedy which influences the course of the disease.[16] Yet prescribing in general practice is the rule rather than the exception.

Quantifying the placebo effect is essential in any rational study of therapy. As Asher has pointed out, the demystification of the placebo effect undermines much of the effectiveness of therapy, and so it is not surprising that authoritarian medicine has an inbuilt resistance to discussing the placebo effect. There are, with a few honourable exceptions, very few placebo controlled trials of therapies commonly used in general practice. Because a pilgrim to Lourdes can no more profit from a discussion with a rationalist than a patient can profit from a lecture on placebos before a placebo is prescribed, the problem of providing informed consent becomes a convenient rationalisation for eschewing trials.

Faith in placebos is advantageous to both doctor and patient; faith in religion to both priest and penitent. Critical enquiry is subversion in one context and blasphemy in the other. Iain Chalmers, who is the Director of the Perinatal Epidemiology Unit at Oxford, introduces his discussion of various authoritarian strategies to prevent enquiry into the placebo effect with these words: 'It is because the scientific method actively fosters uncertainty that it must inevitably be subversive of authority .... If these authorities are to be effective propagandists for their diverse practices and causes, then, unlike scientists, they need the self-confident certainty that they know what is good and what is bad. Searching questions about how they know are only unsettling, they threaten to complicate the simple messages which are such an important component of their work'.[17]

Clearly there is a conflict between the unruffled working of blind faith and admitting ignorance; between the traditional 'art' and the 'science' of medicine. Speaking for authority, Sir Douglas Black, perhaps tempted by the grey landscape of compromise, attempted to diffuse the antithesis between the art and the science of medicine by maintaining that it was a false antithesis.[18] But no compromise is possible. Blau put it bluntly when he said: 'The doctor who fails to have a placebo effect on his patients should become a pathologist or an anaesthetist .... In simple English, if the patient does not feel better for your consultation you are in the wrong game'.[19]

The best way to improve the results of any treatment is to leave out the controls. The doctor benefits, the patient benefits, only science suffers. The spoilsports who insist on controlled trials deprive large numbers of patients of treatments which have hitherto pleased both them and their physicians. For example, Cobb and his colleagues, suspecting that the good results of ligating the internal mammary artery in the treatment of angina pectoris were due to a powerful placebo effect, bravely embarked on a controlled trial.[20] (The internal mammary artery is an artery which runs near the heart and it was suggested that if it were blocked by tying a ligature around it, the blood would be diverted to the heart and that this improved blood supply would relieve the pain of angina). The patients were told that they were participating in an evaluation of this operation but were not told that some of them would undergo a sham operation instead of the real thing. After the surgeon had exposed the artery, a randomly selected envelope was opened which contained an instruction: either ligate or do not ligate. Seventeen patients with angina which was seriously limiting their activities agreed to take part in the study. During the first six months after the operation, 5 out of 8 of the ligated patients and 5 out of 9 of the patients who had had the sham operation were much improved according to their own evaluation. Striking improvement in exercise tolerance occurred in two patients who had had the sham operation.

This trial took place in 1959; a similar trial of coronary artery by-pass surgery today would not be passed by any ethical committee, yet it is certain that some of the apparently good results of such surgery must be due to the placebo effect.

Another group of sceptics repeated the same experiment on 18 patients. Neither the patients nor the cardiologist who assessed the results knew who had had the real operation. 'A marked improvement in the degree of angina occurred in 10 out of the 13 actually ligated. Five patients had a sham procedure and all emphatically described marked improvement.'[21]

Beecher, an American anaesthesiologist and a pioneer research worker into the effects of placebos, noted that immediately after these reports appeared, the operation was dropped, even by those who had previously been its advocates. The life cycle of this placebo operation was only two years, 'a remarkably short time for the introduction and discrediting of a surgical procedure. Significantly, it was destroyed by two or three well-planned double-blind studies.'[22]

It might reasonably be argued that if the operation worked it should not have been abandoned simply because its good results were due to the placebo effect. Its abandonment was justified because the operation was not risk-free; in a larger series it carried a 5% mortality, and predictably it had no effect on longevity. Its good effects were upon the 'illness', rather than on the disease.

The milieu and the placebo, and the Clever Hans phenomenon

The more controlled the conditions and the more sceptical the attitude of the investigator, the less likely a placebo treatment will go unrecognised as such. New drugs create new hopes, and according to advice, variously attributed to Sydenham, Trousseau and Osler, one should treat as many patients as possible with a new drug while it still has the power to heal.

Placebo response rates depend on the milieu in which they are tested. Lowinger and Dobie showed that the nature of the drug tested influenced the placebo response.[23] Elaborate trial rituals, complicated dosage schedules, and the use of what is believed to be a potent drug may increase the placebo response from 25 to 75%.

More recently Gracely and his colleagues studied the effect of a placebo on the pain which follows a dental extraction.[24] It had previously been suggested that the placebo effect on pain was the result of a release of endorphins, morphine - like substances which are produced in the normal nervous system. This hypothesis was based on the observation that naloxone, which is an endorphin antagonist, seemed to reverse the placebo effect on pain.

Life would be simpler if the placebo effect on pain had such a neat and rational explanation. However, subsequent experiments showed that naloxone, in addition to its effect on endorphins, was itself a pain enhancer. Gracely and his colleagues went even further and were able to demonstrate that placebos may in some circumstances increase, rather than decrease, pain depending upon the expectations of those administering the placebo.

They used as subjects patients undergoing extraction of wisdom teeth. The actual study design was complex, but the important findings related to the comparison of two groups of patients who did not know to which of the two groups they had been assigned. They were informed that they would receive injections which *could* relieve pain but might sometimes make it worse. The first group received either placebo or fentanyl, a commonly used pain killer. The study was double blind: that is, neither those administering the injections nor the subjects knew who received fentanyl or who received the placebo. However, the experimenters knew that this part of the study involved a comparison of placebo with fentanyl; as might have been expected, both the active drug and the placebo reduced pain. The second group received either placebo or naloxone and again the experimenters knew the nature of the comparison which was being made. In this instance both the active drug and the placebo *increased* pain!

This apparently paradoxical and surprising finding can only be explained by assuming that those carrying out the experiment indicated their own expectations to the subjects by nonverbal or other means.

This subtle mechanism, which must raise doubts about the validity of many double-blind therapeutic trials, was the subject of a conference on 'The Clever Hans Phenomenon', which was organised by the New York Academy of Sciences in 1981.[25] Clever Hans was a horse belonging to a retired Berlin schoolteacher, who at the beginning of the century astonished the world by demonstrating in the circus ring that Clever Hans could add, subtract, multiply and divide, read and spell and solve problems of musical harmony. It soon transpired that Clever Hans could only perform these astonishing feats in the presence of his master. This apparently extraordinary phenomenon was the result not of remarkable equine intelligence but of Hans' ability to translate subliminal cues from his master into an appropriate number of taps with his hoof.

The Clever Hans phenomenon in double-blind therapeutic trials has been little explored but it is becoming increasingly apparent that double-blinding is difficult to achieve. In a double-blind trial of propranolol against placebo in patients who had recently had a heart attack, nearly 70% of physicians and over 80% of patients correctly guessed which substance had been administered.[26]

The placebo effects of therapeutically active drugs
Another cause of error is to believe that the therapeutic effects of active drugs are always ascribable to their specific pharmacological action. In laboratory experiments using animals or isolated pieces of tissue, the pharmacological effect of a drug can be defined and quantified; however, in clinical use the effect of the drug will depend, not only upon its pharmacology, its chemical composition and its dose but also on the expectations of both doctor and patient, verbal and non-verbal cues and on the patient's conditioning as well as his or her disease.

In his experiments on the effect of suggestion and conditioning on the action of pharmacological agents, Wolf showed that nausea could be stopped by ipecacuanha, a powerful emetic. This was possible provided that the ipecacuanha was given by intragastric tube, so that its bitter taste was not recognised, and that its administration was accompanied by a strong suggestion that it would stop the human guinea pig feeling sick. Concomitant measurement of the contractions of the stomach muscles, normally enhanced by ipecacuanha, showed that in this circumstance they were diminished. Similarly, Wolf's experimental subject, Tom, who had a permanent large gastric fistula, (a channel, the

unfortunate result of previous mishap, which created a direct communication between the stomach and the abdominal wall), was given
prostigmine by mouth on several occasions, always with the same
pharmacologically predictable response - abdominal cramps, diar-
rhoea and local changes in the stomach, hyperaemia, hypersecretion
and hypermotility. Subsequently tap water, if thought by Tom to be
prostigmine, elicited the same response. Even atropine, a pharmacological antidote to prostigmine, would in these circumstances, (when
Tom thought he was being given prostigmine), produce prostigmine-
like effects.[27]

These experiments show that placebo reactions can override pharmacological responses. There are two important consequences of this
understanding. On the one hand, a placebo can imitate a true pharmacological effect, and on the other, the effects of pharmacologically active
substances depend on the setting and the expectations of both patients
and doctors.

The assessment of drugs

As pointed out by Lindahl and Lindwall, the 'real' effect of therapies
cannot be determined from the results of clinical trials because there is
an interaction between the placebo effect and those effects which are
specific to the particular drug. It is quite possible to find that different
double-blind trials of the same treatment produce different results:
sometimes benefit, sometimes harm and sometimes no effect.[28]

The 'real' effects of drugs are confounded by the expectations which
accompany most trials. Such expectations may enhance the good
effects of treatment, an effect which may be further enhanced by
increased medical interest and nursing care. On the other hand the need

to inform patients about the reasons for the trial and present uncertainties are likely to operate in the opposite direction, as is their awareness that decisions about their treatment are being made by the toss of a coin. This is illustrated by healing rates of duodenal ulcer in placebo groups in controlled clinical trials which ranged from 20 to 70%.[29] Finally, the results of such randomised controlled trials may not be same as the effects of the drugs in ordinary clinical practice.

Pain and the placebo response

Misunderstanding about the placebo response in relation to pain is common. Goodwin and his colleagues found that more than half of the house officers and nurses to whom they talked believed that if a patient who was in pain felt better after an injection of sterile water, the pain was 'functional', that is imaginary, and could not have an organic or pathological source.[30] This is to leap from a false premise to a foregone conclusion. Lasagna and colleagues noted that on average three to four out of ten surgical patients suffering from severe wound pain reported satisfactory pain relief after a placebo injection of saline solution.[31] They pointed out that placebo responders are difficult to predict as they are not 'whiners', 'nuisances' or 'young hysterical females' and have the same average intelligence as non-responders. Beecher showed that just as a placebo may or may not elicit an analgesic response, so a wound may or may not evoke pain depending on whether it is construed, among other things, as good or bad. Soldiers wounded in battle may not need an analgesic because their pain is partially relieved by the expectation of being removed from the hell of the front line to a safe hospital and the prospect of being returned to their families. On the other hand similar wounds in civilian life raise questions and anxiety about recovery, financial loss and subsequent disability.

Such observations are not limited to war. A spectacular placebo response was observed by Western delegates during the Great Leap Forward, when Chinese doctors, on the orders of Chairman Mao, discovered acupuncture 'anaesthesia'. Credulous observers believed that the reason Chinese patients did not react to pain was because a needle was being twirled in their ear lobes. They were unaware of many reports, both from China and from Europe, which demonstrated that it was possible for people to bear, in a most stoical fashion, the pain of surgery. In 1843, an American missionary and surgeon, Peter Parker, performed a mastectomy on a Chinese patient, who, when the operation was over, 'raised herself from the table without assistance, jumped upon the floor and made a bow to the gentlemen present, in the Chinese style, and walked into another room as though nothing had occurred.' Another surgeon wrote in 1863 that 'a large proportion of those upon whom operations were performed had no chloroform .... some did not even clench their hands or teeth, but lay upon the table perfectly motionless, while their muscles were being cut by the knife and their bones divided by the saw.' Mitchel, at the beginning of the century, performed amputations, thyroidectomies, mastectomies and other major surgery without general anaesthesia. In Berne in the 1890's, Theodor Kocher carried out 1,600 operations on goitres without general anaesthesia. Harvey Cushing was flabbergasted when in 1900 he witnessed César Roux operating upon the goitres of Valois peasants with no anaesthesia.[32]

Conclusion

The placebo response is a complex phenomenon which is still little understood. The placebo effect contributes to every therapeutic success by helping to alleviate the symptoms of disease, and is often the sole cause of the 'cure' of illness. Since the success and reputation of medicine is based upon its ability to cure, it is perhaps not surprising that doctors refer so seldom to the placebo effect, as the same effect underpins the successes of every charlatan and quack. Considering its essential role in the practice of medicine, the space or time devoted to the placebo in textbooks and lectures for medical students is astonishingly small: a paragraph in a textbook, a hint during a lecture or ward-round. One of the reasons may be that doctors are motivated to deny the importance of the placebo effect, because admitting its potency threatens their image and power.

This chapter alludes only indirectly to those placebo techniques which together are called 'alternative medicine'. This subject is so important that the whole of chapter five is devoted to it.

2

A FISTFUL OF FALLACIES

Introduction

In this chapter we provide some examples of erroneous reasoning, fallacious arguments and faulty logic. These examples are chosen because they seem to us either to be important or not widely recognised. We also explore some of the ways in which truth may be obscured, twisted, or mangled beyond recognition, without any overt intention to do it harm. We are not concerned with deliberate misinformation, deception or fraud, which from time to time pollute the scientific literature; for those that are interested, this scientific 'pornography' has been well reviewed in two recent publications.[1] [2]

Wishful thinking and prejudice, the selective presentation of data, unacknowledged personal bias and self-deception are dangerous disorders because the infection is symptomless and carriers are not immediately recognisable. If we wish to be protected we must become sensitive to subtle signs: slips of the tongue, asides, quasi-religious sentiment disguised by jargon, belief masquerading as established truth.

The fallacy of association being causal

Osler remarked that 'a desire to take medicine is perhaps the great feature which distinguishes man from other animals'. There is another even more important characteristic which distinguishes man from other animals: man's need for explanations. Since time immemorial, doctors and other healers have flourished because neither they nor their patients could distinguish clearly between association and cause and effect. Blood letting and purging, total dental extraction to eliminate 'toxic foci', and irrational polypharmacy have their modern equivalents, because neither doctors nor patients are readily able to distinguish between association and cause. As a result of failing to make this distinction, learning from experience may lead to nothing more than learning to make the same mistakes with increasing confidence. Logicians call this fallacy 'post hoc ergo propter hoc'. I was sick, I am now cured, therefore my treatment was the cause of my recovery.

If there is a relationship between two things or events A and B, this relationship may be of four kinds:

1. A causes B (cause)
2. B causes A (consequence)
3. A and B share a common cause C (collateral)
4. A and B are associated by chance (coincidence)

In our need to understand, to explain, and to treat, the temptation to impute causality to association is pervasive and hard to resist. It is the most important reason for error in medicine.

a. Causal association

When two events are regularly associated, such as smoke and fire, or coitus and pregnancy, it is tempting to regard as logically justifiable the conclusion that the two things are causally related. However, strictly speaking this is a logical nonsequitur. Is life the cause of death because the one always precedes the other? Is night the cause of day, or day the cause of night? Is it sensible to conclude that dogs cause rabbits because rabbits are chased by dogs?

Strictly speaking we can never prove causality from an association, however perfect such an association may appear. In some areas birthrates vary directly with the prevalence of storks. In Dublin, the density of television aerials was strongly associated with birth rate and infant mortality, not because television was lethal to infants but because the density of aerials reflected poor housing, overcrowding and poverty. In the period immediately following the Second World War there was an association between an increased sale of nylon stockings and an increased mortality from lung cancer.

An association, if biologically plausible, may *suggest* a causal link but *proof* is only obtainable by experiment.

b. The unidirectional fallacy

If A is associated with B but precedes B, it still remains possible that B is the cause and not the consequence of A. A feeling of being cold often precedes a febrile illness, but contrary to popular opinion it is not sitting on cold stone benches, walking in wet socks or going out after hairwashing that cause either the feeling of chill or the fever. The feeling of chill is the first symptom of fever.

An association has been described between paracetamol, more commonly known as Panadol, and duodenal ulcers. Many commonly used drugs for the alleviation of pain, such as aspirin, are known to aggravate the symptoms of such ulcers. At first sight it would seem reasonable to conclude that paracetamol also has this effect. There is, however, an alternative possibility, which is the result of advice given to those who have ulcers that they should avoid aspirin and the like, but that they may freely take paracetamol. It is therefore possible that duodenal ulcer 'causes' paracetamol taking, rather than paracetamol 'causes' ulcers.

If withdrawal symptoms follow a period of drug use, it is not the drug but its absence which causes them. This example seems trivial only because we now understand the cause. In the case of an unconscious diabetic patient who is taking insulin, it might be a fatal mistake to presume that because lack of insulin causes coma the proper treatment is insulin. Coma in diabetics may be due to either too little or too much insulin, and since these two states may be difficult to distinguish in the first instance, proper first aid is to administer sugar, because insulin excess is more immediately dangerous and less easily reversible.

c. Collateral or indirect correlation

Since cancer of the uterine cervix is more common in poor people it is perhaps not surprising that one career epidemiologist found a significant association between this cancer and first coitus on the ground rather than in bed.[3]

More seriously, in a debate on an Irish Family Planning Bill, a number of prominent doctors publicly maintained that making condoms freely available would cause an upsurge of promiscuity and venereal disease. Their conviction that there was a causal relationship was based upon an indirect association. In some countries there is an association between the availability of contraceptives and a liberal attitude to sexual activity. But a public demand for readily available contraceptives and a change in sexual behaviour may both be the result of changing societal mores.

d. Necessary and sufficient cause

Even if an association between A and B is causal, it still does not follow that every A will be followed by B. In other words, a necessary cause is not always a sufficient cause. Not everyone exposed to a 'flu virus develops 'flu, therefore exposure to the virus is not itself a sufficient, although a necessary, cause. Not all smokers die of lung cancer and not all people who die of lung cancer are smokers, therefore smoking is neither a necessary nor sufficient cause.

One of Koch's postulates which needs to be fulfilled in establishing the cause of an infectious disease is that a pure culture of the organism, administered to man or animal, must always cause the disease. This seemingly reasonable theoretical requirement does not distinguish between necessary and sufficient cause. That *Vibrio cholerae* is not a sufficient cause of cholera was dramatically demonstrated by Max von Pettenkoffer, the German pioneer hygienist and epidemiologist. In 1892, in full view of an entranced audience, he swallowed 1 millilitre of a fresh culture grown from the stools of a patient who was dying of cholera. He remained unscathed, much to the chagrin of the Kochians. Pettenkoffer did not dispute that the vibrio might be a necessary cause of cholera but he was anxious to prove that it was not a sufficient cause. He may have been expressing a death wish, for nine years later, in his eighty third year, he blew his brains out with a shotgun.

To overcome the difficulty introduced by Pettenkoffer, Koch's postulates were subsequently modified by the rider: 'in susceptible hosts'. This salvage manoeuvre had unforeseen logical consequences. The result was a tautology, since 'susceptibility' depends upon the presence of the disease and 'insusceptibility' on its absence: an organism causes a disease except when it does not.

e. Non-causal time correlation
Among the commonest fallacious associations which occur in epidemi-

ology are those which depend upon a time correlation. Any two independent variables which change linearly over time will show a perfect correlation, an example being the price of beer and the salaries of priests in Chicago.[4] Recently the number of psychiatric inpatients has been plotted against the number of people in prison in England and Wales between 1950 and 1985. This showed a strong negative correlation: as the number of psychiatric inpatients became smaller, the number of prisoners proportionately increased. Although the authors admitted that this association did not necessarily indicate a causal relationship (that is, that those previously admitted to mental hospitals were now being incarcerated in prison), they could not resist concluding that there was 'a compelling reason to doubt the success of community policies, with a reluctance for psychiatrists to admit mentally abnormal offenders'.[5]

Even a perfect correlation does not justify causal inferences if the correlation depends upon comparing two temporal trends. One researcher derived an equation which allowed him to predict lung cancer rates in Australia from petrol consumption between the years 1939 and 1981 and concluded that petrol caused lung cancer.[6] As both lung cancer and petrol consumption were increasing in parallel during this time, the correlation was almost perfect, but this does not justify the conclusion that cars cause lung cancer.

The ecological fallacy
This fallacy stems from transferring relationships which occur in populations to individuals. The ecological fallacy is well illustrated by the hypothetical example of three different populations, each with different incidences of lung cancer and different customs with regard to wearing hats. It is clear that the perfect correlation in the population

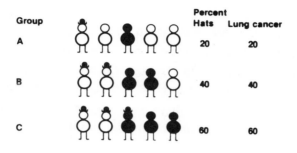

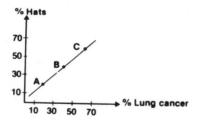

An example of ecological correlation

From: Rosen M, Nystrom L and Wall S:
Guidelines for Regional Mortality Analysis: An Epidemiological
Approach to Health Planning
International Journal of Epidemiology 1985; 14: 293-299

Reproduced by kind permission of the Editor of the
International Journal of Epidemiology

between lung cancer and hat- wearing has no bearing on the likelihood that an individual who wears a hat will develop lung cancer.

Another example is the observation that African natives tend to eat much more fibre than Europeans and have bulkier stools; they also seem to have less of certain diseases which are common in the rich world. This has led Burkitt and others to recommend an alteration in our diet. Similarly, epidemiologists have demonstrated a high positive correlation between national consumption of saturated fats and the incidence of breast cancer. Such evidence does not justify dietary advice to individuals in order to diminish mortality from breast cancer.

This fallacy is of importance in relation to such matters as the prevention of coronary heart disease. Mortality from this disease has been correlated with a large number of variables, which are sometimes different from country to country, and many enthusiasts have been prepared to recommend modifications of diet and life style without the critical experimental evidence. This is so important that we return to it in chapter four.

Intriguingly, there is a strong positive association between mortality in children and the prevalence of doctors in eighteen developed countries.[7] It may be stretching things a bit to advocate a reduction in the number of doctors on the basis of this observation.

Surrogate - outcome fallacy
This fallacy is not as widely recognised as it should be. Since the outcomes or results of medical interventions may be difficult to measure and may be long delayed, there is a temptation to substitute surrogates for real outcomes: a surrogate which can be readily measured within a

reasonable time. Some epidemiologists use the phrase 'intermediate outcomes'. This is less satisfactory because it implies a stage towards the desired outcome rather than a substitution.

Surrogate outcomes should only be used when it is certain that they are valid substitutes for the real outcome. For example, a health education bureau may assess its activity by enumerating the number of leaflets which have been delivered to homes or the amount of television advertising which has been purchased. This surrogate measure does not provide any information as to how many people have changed their behaviour and might, as a result, look forward to better health. A campaign to increase seat-belt wearing in Wessex was shown to have no immediate effects on the number of people using them.[8]

This fallacy is prevalent in screening for disease. The number of women treated following 'positive' smear reports is often used as a surrogate for the real objective, which is a reduction in the number of women dying from cancer of the cervix. As we elaborate later, it is possible to treat increasing numbers of women for 'positive' smears without having any impact on mortality. Similarly the removal of polyps (excrescences of the lining membrane) from the large bowel cannot be accepted as a valid surrogate for diminished mortality from cancer of the colon, although such growths are associated with an increased probability of developing cancer.

A particular form of this fallacy surrounds the increasingly popular activity of audit. Characteristically those who embark on audit set down criteria of performance against which reality is measured. For example, an audit of the management of hypertension might specify, in addition to the measurement of blood pressure, examining the retina and the arteries at the back of the eye with an ophthalmoscope, X-raying the chest to assess the size of the heart, testing urine for protein and undertaking simple blood tests of kidney function. However, such audit does not address an important question: does any of this activity improve the quality of life or diminish the mortality of patients?

The faggot fallacy

American readers may need to be reminded that a faggot this side of the Atlantic is a bundle, usually of sticks, and has nothing to do with sexual orientation. The faggot fallacy is a belief that multiple pieces of evidence, each independently being suspect or weak, provide strong evidence when bundled together. The truth is that a bundle of insecure evidence remains insecure. It has become a fairly common practice to accumulate a number of studies, none of which has demonstrated significant results and by pooling them 'prove' difference. This is a practice which should be regarded with suspicion for two reasons. It is only valid if the individual studies which are 'pooled' are themselves valid. Secondly, it is certain that if large numbers are required to demonstrate a difference, the real difference must be small and therefore likely to be unimportant.

The weight - of - evidence fallacy

This fallacy has much in common with the faggot fallacy. The Popperian approach to science begins from the premise that what distinguishes science from non-science is the possibility of refutation: progress is made by subjecting hypotheses to the most rigorous attempts to prove them wrong. Popper used the example of the black swan: the statement 'all swans are white' is little strengthened by the sight of the thousand and first swan, but destroyed by the sight of one black swan. The only necessary assurance is that the black bird is indeed a swan.

Judging validity by the weight of confirmatory evidence is reminiscent of the tailor whose catch cry was: 'never mind the quality, feel the width'. Weighing evidence in this context is about the accumulation of all evidence which confirms belief on one side of the scales, and showing that its quantity and bulk are greater than the counter-evidence which can be placed upon the other side. Such an approach to establishing truth is non-science: not only is it non-science, it is dangerous because reasoning of this sort may lead to action, which, (particularly in the field of preventive medicine), can touch many people's lives. In the search for truth there is no point in seeking the concordant, in collecting white swans; it is the discordant which offers the possibility of progress towards better understanding.

Unfortunately, there is a temptation to reject the uncomfortable pieces of evidence which do not fit cherished belief. For example the Surgeon General's Report on Smoking cites a very large number of references which support the ill effects of smoking on health but disregards the minority of discrepant data which are not consistent with the conclusions.[9] Yet these are the pieces of evidence which demand the most careful examination. If they are not flawed, the conclusion or hypothesis must be modified to accommodate their findings.

A not uncommon result of this fallacy is the rejection of criticism of popular beliefs as 'selective'. If attention is drawn to, for example, the evidence that nuns may die of cervical cancer, which is in conflict with the view that it is a venereal disease, a common response is that this is the selective use of evidence and ignores the evidence which suggests that promiscuity is important. A more proper response would be a critical examination of the evidence for this cancer in those who have never been sexually active, and if this evidence stands, it should lead to some modification of the original view. The exception destroys the rule.

The Bellman's fallacy

In Lewis Carroll's 'The Hunting of the Snark' the Bellman says: 'What I tell you three times is true'. This is a degenerate form of the faggot fallacy. Waldron identified the Bellman's fallacy in the centuries-old belief that the first mention of lead colic is to be found in the writings of Hippocrates.[10] Several eminent authors of texts on occupational medicine, quoting each other, maintain that Hippocrates was the first to describe the disease. Waldron pointed out that Hippocrates wrote no such thing. Still, since not many prospective authors on lead colic are likely to be familiar with Waldron's letter to *The Lancet* or with the Hippocratic corpus, they will continue to open their learned treatises on lead colic by, 'the first description of lead colic must be accredited to Hippocrates'.

Hamblin debunked the belief that spinach is a rich source of iron by tracing the Popeye-spinach myth to a mistake by the original investigators in the 1930's who put the decimal place in the wrong place and made a ten-fold overestimate of iron content.[11] America was 'strong to finish 'cos they ate their spinach' and many Europeans are still nauseated by the sight and smell of steaming spinach, a reminder of their childhood when their health conscious mothers were force-feeding the stuff to put some iron into their blood. There is more iron in eggs, beef, pork, liver, shellfish, brown sugar and pulse than in spinach, and an equal amount in cabbage, Brussel sprouts and other similar vegetables.

The fallacy of authority

The fallacy of authority is believing things to be true because of the authoritative source of the information. It must be true because I read it in the paper, saw it on television, the surgeon said so, *The Lancet* published it. Authority is deeply rooted in medicine because the patient seeks advice in order to obtain an explanation which is more credible than that of friends and relations.

A respect for authority is the basis for most medical education. Students may become so used to memorising that they become prey to the illusion that the reason for learning to parrot lectures and textbooks is that they are the 'truth'. The most usual answer we receive to the suggestion that students should not believe anything for which the only evidence is the statement of an authority is: 'We have to believe something' and, in loud parentheses, 'we have to pass our examinations'. In our course on the critical appraisal of evidence students are told that if the course is to fulfil its purpose they should leave our department not necessarily believing, without critical examination, those things which we have taught.

Authorities naturally support the status quo, which gives them the right to that accolade. When William Harvey published his discovery of the circulation of the blood he was given the cold shoulder. He complained to his friend Aubrey that after the book came out he lost most of his patients, as it was 'believed by the vulgar that he was crack-brained' and 'all Physicians were against his Opinion, and envied him: many wrote against him'.[12]

There are good reasons for distrusting the opinion of authority, not only in medicine but in science proper. It now sounds incredible that the prestigious scientific journal *Nature* could refuse, on the advice of authorities, to publish Hans Krebs' work on the citric acid cycle, H. C.

Urey's work on heavy hydrogen, and Enrico Fermi's research on beta-decay.[13] Krebs, Urey and Fermi all subsequently received Nobel Prizes for these discoveries. Even more recently, the Nobel Prize laureate Rosalyn Yallow disclosed that '*Science* rejected her communication describing for the first time the principles of radioimmunoassay - a method now used in every hospital laboratory.[14]

Distrusting authority should not be equated with advocating anarchy or with denying the useful role of authority. It may be wise to accept, at least provisionally, what an authority has to say: it is unwise and dangerous to believe. As Wilson Mizner once said: 'I respect faith, but it is doubt that gets you an education.'

One of the best practical tests of the trustworthiness of authorities is to see how they respond to the question: what is your evidence? Thomas Jefferson, the third president of the United States, had this admonition for a young physician: 'His mind must be strong indeed, if, rising above juvenile credulity, it can maintain a wise infidelity against the authority of his instructors, and the bewitching delusion of their theories'.[15]

The more intelligent the authorities, the more idiotic will be some of their claims. This paradox was explained by Francis Bacon (the philosopher, not the painter) who said that when such a man sets out in the wrong direction, his superior skill and swiftness will lead him proportionally further astray.

A classic example of the fallacy of authority is an acceptance of Newton's proofs that the prophecies of the Apocalypse have been fulfilled. In his *Observations upon the Prophecies of Daniel and the Apocalypse of St.*

John, published in 1733, Isaac Newton computed that the Church of Rome became the eleventh horn of the fourth beast of Daniel's vision. By establishing that 'a time and times the dividing time' equals 1260 solar years, Newton predicted the fall of the Papacy between the years 2035 and 2054 (being a good scientist he provided a confidence interval).

Sir William Whitla, MP, MD, DSc, LLD, the Professor of Materia Medica at the Queen's University of Belfast and the Pro-Chancellor of the University, who was also the President of the British Medical Association, and presumably an authority of weight, wrote an introduction to a republication of Newton's *Observations* in 1922. In his introduction he regretted that the manifestations of unbelief, such as scepticism, atheism, agnosticism, materialism and rationalism, were growing. He felt that it was not surprising that among those who dismiss Biblical miracles 'there are still some who deny such modern discoveries as the fact of levitation'! [16]

Fashions in medical treatment are the rule and if they are supported by the voice of authority are difficult to dislodge before they decline into inevitable and tardy death. The *Medical Press* noted in 1900 that: 'During the chequered career of the crusade against consumption many false claims have been noised abroad as to the discovery of this, that or the other infallible cure. The most notorious of these was the tuberculin craze that swept over the whole civilised world about 10 or 11 years ago and was accepted almost universally because it emanated from the illustrious scientist who laid the basis of the scientific treatment of consumption by demonstrating its specific bacillus. Yet Koch's tuberculin proved a snare and delusion'. [17]

Authorities may be as fallible at the end of the twentieth century as at its beginning. In the last ten years many cancer patients have been treated with Vitamin C, mainly on the authority of the double Nobel Prize Laureate, Linus Pauling. A fairly recent well conducted controlled trial showed that Vitamin C not only did not benefit such patients but had a deleterious effect which was significant at the 5% level, that is the odds are only one in twenty that a difference of this magnitude could have occurred by chance.[18] This deleterious effect was, in our view reasonably, ascribed to just such a chance, yet had chance produced a similar result in the opposite direction, Pauling would have been vindicated and no patient would have escaped this, not completely innocuous, treatment.

We should be kind to all people, even those who are vested with authority, but we must be ruthless in seeking and criticising the evidence on which their beliefs are founded.

The fallacy of 'Everybody Says So'

This is a combination of the Faggot Fallacy and the Fallacy of Authority. In the current medical textbooks, two specialty monographs, and also in a standard pharmacopoeia, it is said that phenytoin, a drug commonly used to control fits, can cause red urine, if the urine is acid. Derby and Ward traced this myth to a reference in a pharmacy journal.[19] After telephoning the author they were given the exact source of his reference, which when checked turned out to be without foundation. Derby and Ward were lucky that the myth originated among their contemporaries who were still alive and could be contacted. How much of the clinical 'lore' in textbooks is based on spurious observation which nobody has bothered to check and some of which has been reproduced unchanged from generation to generation? Among the most suspect statements are those about which there is no doubt, where 'everybody says so', but which are not supported by evidence.

Only a few years ago patients who had had myocardial infarcts, (heart attacks), were ordered six weeks absolute bed rest. This was the time adjudged necessary in order to allow the damaged myocardium to heal. Few doctors even allowed the patients to use the commode rather than the bedpan. Those doctors who did so were both eccentric and brave. Now early mobilisation, even within twenty four hours, is the rule and those patients who had been kept in bed for a long time and as a result developed clots in their legs could conceivably sue the doctor for malpractice.

Other fairly recent popular and almost universal beliefs were bland diets for peptic ulcer and low roughage diets for diverticular disease of the colon. Bland diets have been discarded in the treatment of peptic ulcer and *high* roughage is now recommended in diverticulitis.

The fallacy of simple explanation
In their survey of medical bandwagons, Cohen and Rothschild noted that physicians often accept a new idea because it offers a simple solution to a complex problem.[20] But as H.L. Mencken pointed out, 'for every complex problem there is a solution that is simple, direct and wrong'.

Perhaps a better title for this fallacy would be the fallacy of the global explanation. If an explanation is so simple that it explains everything in general, it often explains nothing in particular. Such sweeping explanations and theories are characteristic of alternative medicine. For example, homoeopathy bases all therapeutic activity on one simple principle, the same cures the same, the antecedent of which was the doctrine of brunonianism, first propounded by John Brown, (1735-1788). Brown taught that every disease was either overstimulation (sthenia) or inhibition (asthenia) and that the respective treatments were either opium or alcohol in massive doses. The system was enthusiastically accepted by doctors, and, according to the historian Johann Bass, this treatment was responsible for more deaths than the French Revolution and the Napoleonic Wars combined.

In the last century and at the beginning of this, 'strain' became a popular explanation for many diseases: cardiac strain, sacro-iliac strain, or eye strain which was a major cause of headache. Later on strain was replaced by 'stress', a concept which became extremely popular after Hans Selye made it the centre-piece of his 'general adaptation syndrome'. At present, many doctors, and even more ordinary people, believe that 'stress' causes coronary heart disease, cancer, ulcerative colitis, peptic ulcers and many other disorders. One would have to go back to Galen to find an equivalently grandiose conception, which has no explanatory power but which appears to explain everything.

The magic bullet fallacy

When new drugs are first introduced their introduction is usually accompanied by glowing accounts which stress their effectiveness and their freedom from side effects. Such optimism is falsely grounded because any drug which interferes with the biochemistry of the human organism must have undesirable effects. Experience quickly teaches that the drugs are not as effective as first thought and that their use is by no means trouble free. Only homoeopathic prescriptions are harmless because they cannot have any physical effects, although they may foster delusions of benefit in the psyche.

As David Sackett pointed out, if a side effect occurs on average in one out of every thousand patients, investigators would have to follow three thousand patients to be 95% confident of detecting at least one such occurrence.[21]

The bad-blood fallacy

Quite recently some psychiatrists considered that 'schizophrenia' might be cured by cleansing the blood and removing a schizophrenic 'toxin' by haemodialysis. It is not generally known that this idea first occurred to a schizophrenic patient.[22] Many more diseases of unknown cause have been treated in this way. Blood has mystico-religious connotations and the purity of blood has been part of most reactionary ideologies.

The hypothesis that blood groups might be causally related to various diseases has attractions which are of the global explanation sort. Such notions have a particular appeal for researchers who are somewhat short of ideas. A hypothesis of this kind predicts nothing and prohibits nothing. As there is no reason for hypothesising any particular association, the data on blood groups and diseases may be dredged with a very high probability of finding a 'significant', but nonetheless chance, association. Thus a persistent researcher, who starts with an empty mind, is often rewarded by publishable results. Examples can be found in current and prestigious journals.

In 1962, Alexander S. Wiener, the co-discoverer of the Rh-factor and one of the most eminent forensic scientists, critically reviewed the pseudo-science of associations between blood groups and diseases.[23] Not surprisingly his criticism is seldom referred to by those who continue to churn out such associations. Following his criticism of a claim that there was a 'firm' association between blood group O and duodenal ulcer he was accused of armchair criticism, and it was suggested that the question could only be resolved by the accumulation of more data. His reply is worth quoting: 'This is not necessary, since it has been possible to demonstrate that the data already accumulated, on which the claims are based, are faulty. Moreover, it is not necessary to practice chiropracty in order to demonstrate that chiropracty is a form of quackery: nor is it necessary to try out every crack-brain claim in order to prove such ideas to be fallacious.' Fifteen years later, a *British Medical Journal* editorialist was still expressing surprise that a recent and careful study had found no excess of blood group O in patients with duodenal ulcer.[24]

The fallacy of risk

The fallacy of risk stems from a failure to distinguish between relative and absolute risks. Most of the evidence we have about the possible cause of coronary heart disease and cancers comes from epidemiological studies which express their findings in terms of altered relative risk. The relative risk, although an important index of the strength of an association between a putative risk marker and a disease, has no bearing on the probability that an individual will acquire that disease.

Most aeroplane pilots compared with the rest of us occasional flyers, have *relative* risks of being killed in airline crashes which are probably of the order of thousands to one. Yet neither she nor we should refuse to fly as the *absolute* risk is extremely small.

The futility of taking small relative risks too seriously can be illustrated by a study on smoking, drinking and breast cancer. The researchers showed that alcohol consumption increases the risk of breast cancer less than two-fold, while smoking decreases the risk by half. Yet the researchers did not have the guts to offer the inevitable conclusion to harassed and bewildered women: If you drink, for God's sake, smoke as well! [25]

In a very large study carried out under the auspices of the World Health Organisation in 11 countries, women who had used oral contraceptives for 2-5 years were reported to have a relative risk of 1.5 of developing cervical cancer, as compared with non-users.[26] Leaving aside the researchers' belief that the association was causal, should this be a cause for concern? Fortney et al. analysed the data in terms of life expectancy. The difference in life expectancy between users and non-users, which would be produced by the increased risk of cervical cancer, was 11 days for women aged 20-24 and 7 days for women aged 30-34.[27]

Recently there has been much concern about the possible ill effects of passive smoking. It was stated in parliament that passive smokers were 30% more at risk of lung cancer than others. This illustrates two forms of cheating. Firstly, had this been expressed as a relative risk of 1.3 the effect would have been noticeably less dramatic. Secondly, as Katherine Whitehorn noted in her weekly *Observer* column, this risk, in absolute terms, has moved from 0.09 per 1,000 to 0.12 per 1,000 - a risk increase of less than four hundredths of one per cent. Hardly a proper cause for concern.

Since life itself is a universally fatal sexually transmitted disease, living it to the full demands a balance between reasonable and unreasonable risk. Because this balance is a matter of judgement, dogmatism has little place. Present day preoccupations with health are largely unhealthy as the media constantly draw to our attention hazards to health. Many of these hazards are rare and our individual risk of being harmed extremely small; in this circumstance they should be ignored.

The fallacy of inappropriate extrapolation

Following the Chernobyl disaster many estimates of 'extra deaths' from cancer which might result have been published. These estimations have been based on the assumption that no level of radiation is safe and that it is possible to extrapolate from the effects of high levels of exposure (e.g. Hiroshima and Nagasaki) to low or even very low levels. There is much expert debate about the nature of the relationship between low level radiation and undesirable effects, in particular whether the relationship is linear or non-linear and whether there is a threshold below which no effect occurs.

Richard J. Hickey, a statistician from Pennsylvania, argued that it is conceivable that low levels of radiation could be beneficial; some data from the U.S. and China which correlate mortality and natural back-ground radiation are consistent with this rather surprising notion.[28] Many biological response curves are J-shaped: that is, a little bit of something may be a good thing. Examples are the relationship between alcohol intake and mortality, especially mortality from coronary heart disease, between weight and mortality and possibly between serum cholesterol and death from all causes. Most things - salt, milk, essential metals and even water - are dangerous when taken to excess, but in more appropriate amounts beneficial or essential to health.

Similarly, it is not justifiable to extrapolate from the consequences to health of heavy smoking to the results of smoking five a day. To say that a level of risk, whatever it may be, is equivalent to smoking half a cigarette, or three-quarters of a minute mountain climbing, is an extrapolative nonsense.

The fallacy of the golden mean

This often takes the form of a medical 'consensus conference', which is convened with the express purpose of publishing a statement which represents the consensus view of a panel of experts. In this circumstance one thing at least is certain - no one knows the truth; if they did there would be no need for the conference. Scientific truth is established on the basis of irrefutable evidence, not upon the majority opinion. Nonetheless, reasonableness is believed to lie in moderation happily reposing between extremes. If, for example, some experts claim that standing on one's head prolongs life and another group of equally prestigious experts maintains that this is nonsense, the chairman may well draft a statement, which, needing to be acceptable to both sides, states that: it seems that standing on one's head prolongs life but not as much as was originally claimed. This is a logical non-sequitur: if one extreme view is that 2+2=6, and another is that 2+2=4, it does not follow that to take the moderate view, namely that 2+2=5, is either sensible or safe.

Fallacies in randomised controlled studies

The randomised controlled trial is, despite the difficulties which surround its implementation, the gold standard by which treatments are assessed. The underlying principle is straightforward: people or patients are assigned to two groups by random allocation, that is by chance, by tossing a coin or some other such procedure. One group is designated to receive the new therapy, the other group to receive either no treatment or the accepted management of the day.

Archie Cochrane, whose book *Effectiveness and Efficiency* persuaded many others of the virtues and necessity for the rational assessment of clinical procedures, was the inspiration behind the first brave randomised trial of home versus hospital treatment of heart attacks.[29] He is alleged to have related, though the story may be apocryphal, how some few months into the trial the monitoring group was summoned to receive some disquieting news: there had been eight deaths in the home group as compared with only four deaths in the hospital group. The fears of those who did not believe in the safety of home care were vindicated: it would clearly be unethical to continue the trial. The co-ordinator of the trial suddenly became embarrassed and admitted a mix-up: 'H' in the protocol stood for 'hospital' and not for 'home'. There had been eight deaths in hospital and only four at home. After some moments of awkward silence it was agreed that such small numbers in no way approached conventional levels of statistical significance and that the trial should continue. This is an example of the unethical use of an ethical objection. It is worth noting that neither this trial nor other subsequent similar trials were able to show any advantage of hospital treatment, yet these findings had no effect on the growth and establishment of coronary care units.[30] [31]

Ethical arguments can become an obstacle to scientific enquiry and this is not to be regretted. However, some of the objections could be better described as pseudo-ethical. Chalmers tells of a midwife who wished to assess the effect of routinely administered enemas in women in early labour.[32] She proposed a randomised design but had to fight against the opposition of her colleagues who held that it would be unethical to withold enemas from parturient women. 'The admirable midwife-scientist eventually succeeded in persuading her colleagues to mount the trial, but she had to terminate it earlier than intended'; confronted with the preliminary results suggesting that 'discretionary' enemas are preferable to routine enemas, her colleagues 'turned through 180 degrees and announced that it was now obviously unethical to subject women to routine enemas'.

In the real world it is always difficult and sometimes impossible to carry out randomised controlled trials in a satisfactory manner. Not all prospective double-blind randomised trials are what they pretend to be. Sir Austin Bradford Hill recalled a conversation which ended one such trial. 'Doctor, why did you change my pills?' asked a randomised patient. 'What makes you think that I have?' was the cautious reply. 'Well, last week when I threw them down the loo they floated, this week they sink!'.[33]

The Beethoven fallacy
This is illustrated by an imaginary conversation between two medical colleagues. 'I would like your opinion about a termination of preg- nancy. The father has syphilis and the mother herself has active tuber- culosis. Of the four previous children, the first is blind, the second is dead, the third is deaf and dumb and the fourth has tuberculosis. What would you recommend?' 'I would have no hesitation in recommend- ing termination'. 'Then you would have murdered Beethoven'.

As Medawar points out in discussing this fallacy, unless it is shown that there is some causal connection between syphilis in fathers, tuberculo- sis in mothers and the birth of children who turn out to be geniuses, the world is more likely to be deprived of a Beethoven by chastity than by abortion.[34]

Unfortunately it is on the strength of this sort of argument that abortion referenda are won or lost. One could imagine that some right-wing anti-abortion campaigners, who would not hesitate to use the Beethoven story to support their position, might in other circumstances advocate the sterilisation of 'degenerates'. They would not kill Beethoven because they would not allow his conception.

The Beethoven fallacy has an interesting corollary discovered by H.L.Mencken: 'Because a hundred policemen, or garbage men or bootleggers are manifestly better than one, they absurdly conclude that a hundred Beethovens would be better than one. But this is not true. The actual value of a genius often lies in his very singularity. If there had been a hundred Beethovens, the music of all of them would probably be very little known today, and so its civilising effect would be appreciably less than it is.'[35]

The New-Syndrome fallacy
This is the first of a small selection of statistical fallacies which are pervasive, illuminating or fun. None of them is sophisticated.

Medical literature is full of articles reporting a small number of patients, usually one, who suffer from two uncommon and hitherto unrelated conditions, which are now declared to establish a new 'syndrome', with the tacit hope that it will become eponymously known by the describer's name. The fallacy rests on the assumption that if both conditions are rare, say with a prevalence of 1 in 1000 each, their simultaneous occurrence has a probability of 1 in 1,000,000 and therefore extremely unlikely to be due to chance. The multiplication of the individual probabilities is only permissible if the two conditions were named before the observation had been made. There is nothing improbable in drawing any number from a box which contains pieces of paper with all numbers from 1 to 1,000,000. However, if we drew a number which appealed to us, e.g. our birth date or 1,000 or 10,000, we would be much more impressed than if we drew 8543 or 18311. One of the reasons that some people expect the end of the world in the year 2000 is their belief that God, like the World Health Organisation, thinks in round numbers.

An event should not be considered as having special significance because it is unlikely. As William Silverman reminded us, the probability of being dealt thirteen spades, or any other previously predicted hand, is 1 in 653,013,559,600. The fact that to the bridge player thirteen spades has more meaning than an ordinary hand obscures the reality that the probability of being dealt any other previously unpredicted hand is exactly the same. Bertrand Russell illustrated this point by referring to the licence numbers of passing cars: the prior probability of seeing any particular named number is similar to the probability of many a miracle.

Common sense is a laudable attribute but it cannot stand as substitute for critical and logical thinking. The deceiving potential of common sense can be illustrated by the birthday fallacy. Imagine a party of 23 randomly selected people. What is the probability that at least two of them share the same birthday? It is an astonishing one in two! If the number of people is increased to 47, the probability of two of them having the same birthday is 0.95; in other words, if you use this as a party trick it will work 19 times out of 20. With 57 people the probability increases to 0.99, and with 70 people to 0.999.

The fallacy of insignificant significance
Clinicians reading medical literature are tempted to equate statistical significance with clinical importance, forgetting that statistical significance is a *probability* statement (the likelihood of rejecting the null hypothesis if true) and has nothing to do with the *magnitude* of a

measured difference. If large numbers of patients are required to show benefit from a treatment, it is certain that the treatment is marginal and it is probable that it is of no practical importance.

Large studies often involve a number of centres or, what is even less desirable, the pooling of results. Such studies have been particularly common in assessing new treatments for myocardial infarction or cancer. They are justified by arguing that these are such common and serious conditions that even a small improvement will better the lot of a large number of patients. This justification is largely spurious, because the chance of an individual benefiting is small and most of the treatments carry a burden of side effects, invasive procedures, or other nastiness.

The other sort of study in which large numbers may often be involved is the case-control study. When the groups are large, differences in terms of *relative* risk may often be statistically significant but of no importance in terms of an alteration in *absolute* risk. Small differences in large studies should also be regarded with suspicion because of the many sorts of bias which may afflict such studies. On the other hand, large differences in small studies run the risk of being disregarded if the differences are not statistically significant. This is technically known as a Type 2 error.

The fallacy of post-hoc statistics
It is quite common in the medical literature to see 'p' values attached to differences, which have been noticed in the analysis of data but which were not related to the original hypothesis which the study set out to test. A 'p' value is an estimate of the likelihood that the differences which have been observed could have occurred by chance alone. When

'p' values are small, less than one in twenty or one in a hundred, it is often assumed that the differences must be real. Differences which are discovered by accident then become the verification of an ad-hoc hypothesis which was the result of the observation. This is fallacious because it confuses pre- and post-test probabilities.

As Bailar pointed out, this common fallacy cannot quite be called lying, although such reporting is potentially, and occasionally deliberately, deceptive. 'It is widely recognised that t-tests, chi-square tests, and other statistical tests provide a basis for probability statements only when the hypothesis is fully developed before the data are examined in any way. If even the briefest glance at a study's results moves the investigator to consider a hypothesis not formulated before the study was started, that glance destroys the probability value of the evidence at hand .... When either the (statistical) test itself or the reporting of the test is motivated by the data, a probability statement such as " 'p' less than 0.05" is deceptive.' [36]

The fallacy of 'positive' results

This is also known as a Type 1 error: that is, finding a significant difference between groups due to sampling variation, when in fact there is no real difference between the populations studied. Such results are more likely to be published than negative findings. If, for example, ten research groups in ten different centres study a new and exciting treatment for schizophrenia, the results might be of this kind. Six groups find no demonstrable effect, two find at least a suggestion of a deleterious effect, and two demonstrate some degree of benefit. If one had the opportunity to read all these studies it would be reasonable to conclude that the treatment was worthless. Unfortunately, the studies which are most likely to be published are those which show a 'positive' effect.

The eight groups who did not find what they had expected may convince themselves that the reason that they were unable to demonstrate the expected effect was a Type 2 error - falsely accepting that there was no difference. On the other hand, those whose results are in 'the right direction' are likely to submit a paper to a specialty journal, and if the editor is an enthusiast for the hypothesis which provides a rationale for the treatment, he will almost certainly have it published. Type 1 errors are more serious than Type 2 errors because it is more difficult to publish a refutation, a 'negative' result, than to correct an error which is the result of studying a small sample.[37]

Error of the third degree
This term was coined by Robert Schlaifer to describe the misapplication of statistical procedures. Statistical significance has become the yardstick by which treatments and many other things are evaluated, yet relatively few physicians are statistically sophisticated. As a result the use of an inappropriate statistical method may demonstrate difference where none exists. This is not uncommon, even in the best of journals, and such sins may sometimes be committed by statisticians themselves.[38]

As Alvan Feinstein, one of the greatest American epidemiologists, has noted: 'Some of the major intellectual maladies of modern medical literature arise from the inappropriate extension of statistical significance.'[39] Or as Disraeli falsely put it: 'there are three kinds of lies: lies, damned lies, and statistics.'

The fallacy of obfuscation

Language may illuminate or obscure. It can hide ignorance or expose the facts. It can keep knowledge esoteric and so be an instrument of power, or it can make knowledge available to everyman and thereby undermine power. In medical writing, we should strive for clarity. This is not a matter of style, which is an aesthetic concept, although most clear writing is aesthetically pleasing. Tortuous verbosity may be mistaken by the naive for erudition. Take for example this sentence from *The New England Journal of Medicine*: 'Declining lactation performance, as it is occurring in periurban areas in developing countries, has a community anti-contraceptive effect, increasing the birth rate, and hence the population pressure.' Translated, the sentence means: the decline of breast feeding in shanty towns increases the birth rate. Verbiage may hide manipulation of data. For example: 'Exploratory estimates yielded extreme values on some of the parameters. However, closer scrutiny of the original data suggested that, in all probability, some of the data was from a divergent sample. After discarding the heterogeneous data, logically consistent and statistically significant values and correlations were obtained.' This translated means: 'we threw out what did not fit.'

Short words may also be abused. In 1812 the editor of the *Medical and Physical Journal* wrote: 'Pithed is a barbarism foisted into philosophical debates by some unknown or obscure experimenter on animal life. It is now only intelligible by a periphrasis, and future generations will hardly know it as synonymous with killing.'[40] Nowadays experimental animals are neither pithed or killed, they are 'sacrificed'. To which God, authors never say. Even poor cells can become immolated victims on the altar of science: 'The cells were then sacrificed for electron-microscopic examination.'[41]

Tautology may sometimes pass for knowledge. Asher recalled a viva at which the following dialogue took place: 'What is the vitamin preventing scurvy?' 'Vitamin C'. 'And what is the vitamin?' 'Ascorbic acid'. This satisfied the examiner but Asher noted that what was said amounted to stating that the substance preventing scurvy was a substance preventing scurvy, known as anti-scurvy, that is a-scorbic acid.[42]

Houston and Swischuk proposed to abandon the terms genu valgum, genu varum, talipes equinovarus, hallux valgus and cubitus valgus, since varus and valgus are ambiguous and interchangeable. 'Bow legged', 'knock-kneed', 'club foot', 'bunion' and 'increased carrying angle', are preferable not only because they are less ambiguous, but because the patient can understand them.[43]

Euphemisms disguise unacceptable reality. In a recent communication to the *New England Journal of Medicine*, a young surgeon who had died of AIDS was described as 'a member of a group at increased risk of AIDS'. From the context it appears that he was neither a Haitian nor a haemophiliac. This in a country where homosexuality was declared 'not a disease' by a vote of the American Psychiatric Association.

The 'learning curve' is a euphemism for the phenomenon that with experience and practice the harm done to patients by surgery or invasive procedures diminishes. It disguises the reality that some patients succumb, not to their disease, but to the fumblings of trainees gaining experience, or of a team learning a new procedure. *A barba de necio aprenden todos a rapar* (all learn to shave on a fool's chin).

'Uncompensated care' refers to the absence of care for those citizens of the United States who do not have health insurance or who have less than comprehensive protection. 'Less developed countries' and 'social class V' mean poor countries and poor people.

In conversations which take place in the presence of the patient, 'supratentorial' replaces 'imaginary', or 'in the head'. 'Functional' diseases are those for which no 'real' explanation is found. In the past such patients were known as neurotics or neurasthenics, and if they were women, hysterical. According to one acute observer, 'anybody who enjoys women and tobacco, who is charitable or excitable, is neurasthenic.'[44]

The fallacy of covert bias
It is relatively easy by careful reading of most scientific articles to discover the direction in which the authors would wish to see the results going, and thus to be alerted to the possibility that the results were pushed in that direction. Further evidence derives from the kind of references quoted - selective use of evidence - and from the kind of data and references not quoted - selective use of results; from the choice of vocabulary; from the way in which conflicting data, the author's own and that of others, are discussed or dismissed; and from the source of sponsorship or financing.

Martin compared phrases in two articles on the effect of supersonic transport on the stratospheric ozone layer:[45]

Johnson (*Science*)	Goldsmith et al. (*Nature*)
ozone shield	ozone layer
burden of nitrous oxide	amount of nitrous oxide
threat to stratospheric ozone layer	interact with, and so attenuate the ozone layer
permitting harsh radiation to penetrate the lower atmosphere	radiation reaching the planetary surface

It is clear from these few comparisons that Johnson believes that the problem in question poses danger, while Goldsmith is neutral.

Martin gives the following list of strategies used by scientists when faced with data which do not fit their preconceived theories:

1. flat denial
2. scepticism about the source of the item
3. ascription of an ulterior motive to the source
4. isolation of the item from its context
5. minimalisation of the importance of the item
6. interpretation of the item to suit one's purpose
7. misunderstanding of the item
8. thinking away or just forgetting the item.

Bertrand Russell pointed out: 'Even a learned scientific article about the effects of alcohol on the nervous system will generally betray by internal evidence whether the author is or is not a teetotaller; in either case he has a tendency to see the facts in the way that would justify his own practice.'[46] In this we ourselves are inevitably guilty. Those who can read between the lines may come to know us better than we know ourselves.

The 'Gold Effect' fallacy

Beware the 'Gold Effect', described by Professor T. Gold in 1979.[47] At the beginning a few people arrive at a state of near belief in some idea. A meeting is held to discuss the pros and cons of the idea. More people favouring the idea than those disinterested will be present. A representative committee will be nominated to prepare a collective volume to propagate and foster interest in the idea. The totality of resulting articles based on the idea will appear to show an increasing consensus.

A specialised journal will be launched. Only orthodox or near orthodox articles will pass the referees and the editor.

This effect would be observed even if there were no deliberate selection of believers in the subsequent steps. In reality, the human frailty of scientists augments the whole process. Once the idea penetrates into 'reputable journals' it becomes difficult to eradicate, since most of the readers are innocent-minded and find it unnatural to doubt 'authorities'. 'With the eye of faith, they absorb it at their own level, and pass it on as gospel to others'. The gregarious instinct will also tend to draw together people that entertain the same 'beliefs' and who need to belong. Articles on the idea, initially starting with 'evidence has accumulated', rapidly move to articles which open 'The generally accepted', and before long to 'it is well-established', and finally to 'it is self-evident that'.

The club of believers refuse to enter into discussion with their detractors, who are generally branded as hypercritical paranoiacs, nitpickers and irrationalists. The Gold effect is further accelerated by a glut of publications 'confirming' the idea, since young researchers, eager to have some publications on their next job application, are encouraged to submit papers paying lip-service to the dogma; papers which are much more likely to be accepted by the the club editors than articles showing defects in the official theory or which take the theory head-on. The Gold effect has been particularly noticeable in consensus statements such as those regarding the role of diet in the cause of ischaemic heart disease. Such statements lay little stress on the absence of good experimental evidence or on the existence of discordant data.

The 'hush, hush' fallacy

Hilfiker, a family doctor in rural Washington, confessed publicly in a moving article to some of his professional mistakes, which included a wrong diagnosis of miscarriage, which led to the dilatation and curettage of a uterus containing a 13 week old foetus.[48] The reason for the error was easy to understand with hindsight: the patient had had repeatedly negative pregnancy tests and reliance on false-negative tests had led to the tragedy. 'To my hands, the uterus now seemed bigger than it had two days previously, but since all the pregnancy tests were negative, the uterus couldn't have grown.'

Some correspondents reacting to this article were 'appalled' and 'shocked'. This reaction is typical of authoritarian hypocrisy. Practising physicians have to make large numbers of daily decisions on the basis of incomplete information and ignorance; mistakes, some of them with serious consequences, are inevitable. Since the consequences of medical error may have dramatic results, there is a strong tendency to deny them: the good physician does not make mistakes.

McIntyre and Popper showed that this attitude is linked to the non-scientific nature of medicine.[49] In science, mistakes are inevitable, since science rests on conjecture and hypothesis, trial and error. Medicine, on the contrary, rests on an authoritarian tradition: truth is vested in authority. 'An authority is not expected to err, if he does his errors tend to be covered up to uphold the idea of authority. Thus, the old ethics lead to intellectual dishonesty. This leads us to hide our mistake, and the consequence of this tendency may be worse even than those of the mistake that is being hidden. They influence our educational system which encourages the accumulation of knowledge and its regurgitation at examination. Students are punished for mistakes. Thus they hide ignorance instead of revealing it'. Moreover, as Hilfiker pointed out 'the climate of medical school and residency training ..... makes it nearly impossible to confront the emotional consequences of mistakes........ Since there has been no permission to address the issue openly, I lapse into neurotic behaviour to deal with my anxiety and guilt. Little wonder that physicians are accused of having a God complex; little wonder that we are defensive about our judgements, little wonder that we blame the patient or the previous physician when things go wrong, that we yell at the nurses for their mistakes, that we have such high rates of alcoholism, drug addiction and suicide.'[48]

The fallacy of experience

Featherstone, Beitman and Irby illustrated the distortion of learning from a single experience.[50] A doctor attempted an invasive diagnostic procedure and the patient developed an unusual complication and died. After this the doctor became very reluctant to use the procedure despite the fact that it had been shown to be a low-risk investigation and presumably of diagnostic value.

A geriatric patient with a positive cancer screen refused to have further tests and later was found to have advanced cancer. The doctor was criti-cised by his colleagues and now pushes all patients into extensive evaluation of all abnormal tests.

A resident doctor achieved a high reputation by diagnosing a rare disorder. The diagnosis was first ridiculed by the attending physicians but confirmed by surgery. The resident was highly praised. Since then he has continued to make the same diagnosis in similar patients, wrong in each case and leading to unnecessary interventions.

A physician observing a good remission in advanced cancer after a course of toxic chemotherapy now uses the same treatment for all cancer patients regardless of consequences. On the other hand, a nasty side effect, if part of one's own experience, is a much more powerful disincentive to using that drug than any statement of statistical probability in its favour.

These are examples of the abductive inference, to use the term coined by the philosopher, C.S.Pierce. Abduction is the elementary form of induction, generalising from a very small number of instances, often only one. Although it is a reasoned guess, it is nearly always wrong. There are, however, exceptions, as the linguist Peter Maher said: 'It is healthy to generalise from a single experience that a charging elephant is dangerous to the law that charging elephants are dangerous. One might later - when the danger is past - expand the statistical sample.'[51]

Clinicians are well known for their anecdotes and horror stories. Such tales enliven a lecture or teaching round. 'The last case like this had ...'or 'in my experience..' should always be supplemented by an objective assessment of the prior probability and true frequency of such occurrences, based on reliable independent sources. Personal experience can never serve as a substitute for critical appraisal, good data and sound experiment.

3

DIAGNOSIS AND LABELLING

Introduction

While those who use alternative therapies are generally more concerned with their patter than with accurate diagnosis, teachers in medical schools constantly stress the importance of diagnosis. Diagnosis is the basis for appropriate treatment and sometimes it is pursued for its own sake. From the patient's point of view it may also provide much needed reassurance by demystifying the unknown or by justifying a benign prognosis.

Unfortunately diagnosis, the disease label, has other important and undesirable consequences. Firstly - the disease label transfers people to a new category, that of patient. This often reduces their autonomy. The label also mandates and legitimises doctor interference, which may not always be beneficial. It also offers the possibility of taking up the 'sick role' and so escaping ordinary social obligations, something which may readily become a way of life. Lastly, being diseased is abnormal: it is a form of deviance which may diminish employability, desirability, and marriage prospects or even lead to limitation of liberty by being placed in institutional care or even committed to prison. It follows that diagnosis has a potential for harm as well as for good and that diagnostic error or false labelling is a serious matter.

The diagnostic process

The most popular recent view is that diagnosis is achieved by the use of a hypothetico-deductive method.[1][2][3] This postulates that in the first few moments of a new consultation physicians begin to 'generate' diagnostic 'hypotheses'. As often happens, long words hide trivial concepts. 'Hypotheses' are informed guesses, similar to those generated by the mechanic when faced with the symptoms of a malfunctioning car. Doctors' guesses derive from the age and sex of the patient, from the context, and the specialty of the doctor. Macartney, a paediatric cardiologist, has stressed the importance of prior probability in the diagnostic process; that is, the likelihood of a particular disease being present.[4] Sudden headache and vomiting in an 80-year-old is unlikely to be migraine; a routine attendance at outpatients is unlikely to be an emergency; multiple sclerosis improbable in the gastroenterology clinic. One of us has argued that to dignify these notions as hypotheses devalues the word, although it gives a quasi-respectable 'scientific' appearance to something which is much more pedestrian.[5]

Sackett and his colleagues have used 'Auntie Minnie' as shorthand for recognition which ensures that we seldom slap surprised strangers on the back and enables us to attach labels with confidence to some skin diseases, some strange appearances, and some deformities.[1] Recognition extends far beyond those abnormalities which are identifiable by sight; usually the first few words of a consultation immediately raise the thought 'this sounds like'. 'This sounds like' is based upon knowledge and experience - knowledge of probability and the experience of having seen it before. As a general rule, the presence of physical disease and its probable nature are identified within a matter of minutes and confirmation is sought by selective examination or simple investigation. In practice, symptoms are often simple; a sore throat speedily, and properly, leads to having a look, and any attempt by a young physician to undertake a systems review, or to enquire about drinking habits or the date of the last period will be rightly resented. In outpatients, examining the lump in the groin takes precedence over protracted history taking, and the decision to carry out endoscopy (passing a flexible telescope from the mouth into the stomach and duodenum) to confirm a suspected ulcer is not postponed until other diagnostic possibilities have been explored.

The need for diagnosis

Physicians often maintain that patients are unhappy if they do not receive an explanation for their symptoms, a label, a diagnosis. This inevitably leads to diagnoses which have no firm basis. Since the time of Sir James Mackenzie, honest general practitioners have admitted that in only a minority of new presentations can they make a diagnosis which explains, as distinct from describes, the patient's discomfort. The effects of denying the patient a label have been studied by K.B.Thomas in a series of publications.[6][7] In his 1978 study, 200 patients in whom no definite diagnosis could be made were either given a symptomatic diagnosis and medication, or they were told that they had no evidence of disease and therefore required no treatment. No difference in outcome was found. In his 1987 study he looked at the effect of consultations carried out in either a 'positive' or 'negative' manner. In the 'positive' consultations the patient was given a confident diagnosis and firm reassurance, in the 'negative' consultations the patient was told ' I cannot be certain what is the matter with you'. Whether or not treatment was provided made no difference to the outcome. On the other hand, 64 % of those managed 'positively', as compared with only 39% of those managed 'negatively', reported that they had 'got better'. It seems that a confident approach by the physician who does not admit to any doubts is therapeutically useful, and that this effect is independent of a diagnostic label or treatment with pills.

Benefits of diagnosis

The most obvious benefit of a diagnosis which is firmly based is that it is likely to lead to a sensible management plan which may include appropriate therapy. This is the reason that diagnosis and diagnostic skills are seen to be preeminently important in medical education. The second obvious benefit is that it provides a basis for prognosis. It is diagnosis which predicts the future, be it recovery or death.

A benign diagnosis is a very important part of reassurance. Pain which does not have an obvious and recognisable cause needs to be explained. It is more often this need for explanation than the severity of pain which leads people to seek professional help. A simple and benign diagnosis or explanation provides powerful and effective reassurance. 'It is only a slight strain, there is no question of arthritis'.

Sick role

A less well recognised benefit of a diagnostic label is legitimisation of the sick role. It was an American sociologist, Talcott Parsons, who first drew attention to the fact that in our society there is only one acceptable way to escape our social obligations and that is to be allowed to take up the role of being sick. Only by being sick can we escape going to work, going to school, washing dishes, going to parties or having sexual intercourse. He pointed out that society places conditions on those who wish to be sick. Firstly, they must behave sick. If we complain of being unwell we may be sent to bed with hot water bottles, aspirin and concern. When we awake we may expect to be faced with Bovril and a cream cracker. Having dinner is conditional on taking a share of the washing up. It is not possible to be sick and play golf. In addition to behaving sick, those who want to be sick must express the wish to be well and after a few days to seek professional help. For this reason doctors are involved in legitimising the statement: 'I am sick and therefore I cannot ..... '. For this purpose it may sometimes be necessary to provide a certificate, duly authenticated, but it may be sufficient to be 'attending the hospital', or to be 'under the doctor'. For many house-wives the 'bottle of pills' provides the equivalent of certified sick status and many repeat prescriptions may be necessary to this end. Because being sick allows people to manipulate their environment to what appears to be their advantage, many people come to doctors, not to be made well, but to be kept sick. Finally it is difficult to be convincingly sick without a diagnostic label; once such a label has been acquired it may become a precious necessity and woe betide the doctor who tries to take it away.

Diagnostic error
The first reason for error is ignorance. Doctors can only diagnose diseases that they know and that are within their ordinary terms of reference. This is why new diseases are, after their first description, seen everywhere - AIDS, for example. Ignorance is also the reason that general practitioners may fail to diagnose uncommon conditions. If the physician is unaware that a certain constellation of symptoms and signs indicates a particular disease, there is no possibility of that diagnosis being reached; the diagnosis was missed because it was not considered. The apparent diagnostic acumen of the senior clinician may be nothing more than 'déjà vu'; having seen it before, he can now recognise it. Experience may up to a point protect against diagnostic error by enabling doctors to recognise those pieces of information that are odd or discordant and ring warning bells that things may not be what they

seem.

Although knowledge and experience are the mainstay of diagnostic skill, over-reliance on their virtues frequently leads to nothing more than making the same mistakes with increasing confidence.

Levels of diagnosis

The statement that this patient has a sore throat is one level of diagnosis. This can be made more precise by describing the part of the throat which is affected and then calling it tonsillitis, pharyngitis or laryngitis. Alternatively the discovery of enlarged glands in the armpits and groins in a young adult may lead to a provisional diagnosis of glandular fever. Diagnosis may be further refined by identifying the responsible organism, streptococcal sore throat for example, and determining the organism's susceptibility to various antibiotics.

Generally diagnosis is not pursued further than is necessary to initiate a management plan. This may involve attempts to measure the extent and severity of disease but as a rule does not explain why *this* person contracted *this* disease at *this* particular time.

Diagnosis in psychological and social terms

General practice in particular stresses diagnosis in psychological and social terms. Emphasis on the psychological and social context of symptoms and diseases is not only appropriate but essential if doctors are to help patients. Failure to recognise the social and cultural milieu in which the symptoms are set may lead to inappropriate advice or inadequate reassurance. This may be unimportant when speedy and effective treatments are available. If, on the other hand, the disease is chronic or incurable, treating the disease and ignoring the person who is suffering is bad medicine. Not surprisingly those who have been the victims of such 'treatment' may seek help elsewhere. It is natural that sick people are worried, anxious, and often depressed, but it is unhelpful to call this 'psychological' diagnosis. Similarly 'social diagnosis' is a misnomer for recognising that lack of home, job, money or lover, may contribute to disease and delay and impede recovery.

Physical disease
Diseases which do not have names do not exist. Doctors can only diagnose conditions which have been described. A previously nameless disease only becomes 'real' after its new name has been bestowed upon it. It is less obvious that diseases which have a name may not exist. Mill in *A System of Logic* put it as follows: 'Mankind in all ages has had a strong propensity to conclude that wherever there is a name, there must be a distinguishable separate entity corresponding to the name: and every complex idea which the mind had formed for itself by operating upon its conceptions of individual things, was considered to have an outward objective reality answering to it.'

The belief that words have a meaning of their own is a relic of word magic. As Locke has it: 'Words in their primary or immediate signification stand for nothing but the ideas in the mind of him who uses them'. Diagnosing 'non-disease' is more common than missing the diagnosis of a disease which is actually present. As T.J.Scheff pointed out, by their training doctors are encouraged to err on the side of caution.[8] The most serious 'crime' in the teaching hospital is a missed diagnosis. The greatest credit surrounds an obscure diagnosis achieved by unusual perspicacity or simple good luck. Such successes are subsequently the subject of grand rounds or, not infrequently, death conferences. In other words, doctors are encouraged to commit a Type 1 error, creating a non-disease, rather than a Type 2 error, missing a true disease. When in doubt, diagnose. A Type 1 error convicts the innocent, a Type 2 error acquits the guilty. The commonest disease, in Karl Kraus' aphorism, is diagnosis.

The advantages and disadvantages of these two sorts of error can be summarised:

Consequences of a Type 1 error (disease absent but diagnosed)
1.Unnecessary treatment, which may include surgery.
2. Diminished perception of health and encouragement to become sick.
3. There is almost no risk of incurring opprobrium or of being sued. (The possibility of a legal action for 'defamation of health' should perhaps be encouraged).
4. Correcting this sort of error is unusual and difficult. Sometimes the evidence is destroyed; for example, non-tumours may be washed down the sluice.

Consequences of a Type 2 error (disease present but not diagnosed)
1. A legal action for negligence.
2. Moral condemnation and opprobrium from colleagues BUT
3. The error may be corrected when the disease becomes more florid and more readily apparent.

Non-disease
Considering its importance the literature on non-disease is surprisingly sparse. However, Meador has classified non-diseases into the following seven categories.[9]
1. Mimicking syndrome: e.g. non-Addison's disease (pigmentation and 'low' blood pressure in the absence of abnormality of hormone secre-

tion from the adrenal gland).

2. Upper-lower limit syndrome: (e.g. wrong diagnosis based on spurious borderline laboratory findings).

3. Normal variation syndrome: (e.g. non-dwarfism in familial short stature).

4. Laboratory error syndrome: (e.g. John Smith who lives in Beckenham being treated as John Smith who lives in Dulwich).

5. Radiological over-interpretation syndrome: (e.g. a tumour seen on an X-ray but no tumour found at surgery).

6. Congenitally-absent-organ syndrome: (e.g. 'nonfunctioning kidney' on X-ray; absent kidney at surgery).

7. Over-interpretation-of-physical-findings syndrome: (e.g. non-hepatomegaly when the liver is displaced downwards rather than enlarged).

Dudley Hart, that most sensible of rheumatologists, has suggested the following classification:

1. Anatomical non-disease: normal variation of human shapes and forms, bat ears, winged shoulder blades ('your little angel is growing wings'), non-scoliosis (scoliosis is a curvature of the spine sometimes detected at routine examination carried out by school doctors; most of the children have 'schooliosis' rather than a disease).

2. Clinical non-disease: cardiac non-disease in schoolchildren, non-hypertension due to nervousness on the consulting room couch, non-myxoedema (deficiency of thyroid hormone) in old people with husky voices, hairless bodies, constipation and cold intolerance; a common sign reported by housemen is 'early clubbing', that is, normal curvature of the nails; consultants also have their pet disorders.

3. Investigational non-disease: high levels of blood uric acid in non-gout (they also occur in real gout), the ascription of symptoms to the

coincidental finding of an extra cervical rib, or a narrowed disc space on X-ray (thus creating non-cervical rib disease and non-disc disease), non-hypoglycaemia diagnosed on the basis of a relatively low blood sugar found in a single specimen.

4. Pharmacological non-disease: non-drug-side-effects after adverse media reports.

5. Psychiatric non-disease.[10] (Such a major issue that it rates separate consideration later in this chapter).

A good example of the radiological over-interpretation syndrome comes from a study of 14,867 chest films taken to identify tuberculosis.[11] 1,216 were falsely positive, that is 8.2%, whereas only 24 were falsely negative. Perhaps in this instance it is better to be safe than sorry, but false positives bring with them a burden of unnecessary anxiety and further tests.

A common, and until recently not well recognised, non-disease is preputial adhesions in small boys. It is difficult to imagine the heap of foreskins which have been sacrificed to this imaginary disorder.

Gross has described a prevalent non-cardiac syndrome under the name of the 'emperor's clothes syndrome'.[12] The incidence is highest in the middle grades of training. The epidemiology definitely favours Coronary Care Units, rounds and specialist clinics as high risk areas. The prestige and dominance of the carrier is a major factor in the spread of the disease. In a typical non-cardiac syndrome the chief is making his rounds in the unit with four residents and three interns. He listens and hears a murmur. Nobody else hears it, but after the senior resident says: 'I hear it', the setting is perfect for a mini-epidemic. Down the line, in rapid succession, members of the group are infected. The diagnosis can easily be made by the pathognomonic sign, 'I hear it'. Here *formes frustes* are common, especially in the higher grades of training. The diagnosis is made by saying 'it's very soft', 'it's intermittent' or 'it can only be heard in the saggital decubitus' (which may mean lying on one's side or perhaps lying on one's back).

While a number of studies have examined inter-observer and intra-observer variation in the interpretation of such tests as X-rays and ECGs, relatively little attention has been paid to the reliability of physical signs. It seems probable that such signs as a collapsing pulse, the ability to detect 'the dorsalis pedis' (a pulse felt on the top of the foot) or a minor degree of dullness to percussion, would demonstrate considerable variability.

When non-disease reaches epidemic proportions, the matter can be serious. Weinstein and Stamm described twenty hospital infection non-epidemics investigated by the Center for Disease Control in Atlanta.[13] They included non-epidemics of bacteraemia, respiratory-tract infection, gastroenteritis, skin infections, halothane-induced hepatitis, neonatal jaundice, meningitis and tuberculosis. The causes were errors in specimen processing, contamination of specimens and poor clinical judgement.

Perhaps the most serious non-epidemic was the swine non-flu in the USA in 1976. Forty six million people were vaccinated before the swine influenza programme was halted and, as a direct consequence of the vaccination, some of them died. No swine 'flu appeared and the Director of the Center for Disease Control was sacked.[14]

Koro

In 1975 Agence France-Presse disseminated the following report: 'Rumours that the eating of tunny fish is responsible for a disease which causes the sex organ to wither have caused a slump in the fish trade in the Sumatran port of Palem Bang'.

The disease in question is 'koro', a Javanese word for the head of the turtle, a particularly intriguing, and certainly distressing, non-disease. The disease is popular in Malaysia and in South China, where it is known as 'suck young' or Shook Yang, 'Shrinking penis'. According to the local experts who held a seminar during a koro epidemic in 1967, the disease is due to fear, rumour-mongering, climatic conditions and imbalance between heart and kidney.[15] Patients afflicted by this dreadful malady live in mortal fear of dying and try to prevent the final disappearance of the penis into the abdomen by holding it with 'clamps, chopsticks, clothes pegs etc.', even a 'safety pin'. In some instances the relatives take turns 'to hold on to the penis', and sometimes the wife is asked to keep the penis in her mouth to reduce the patient's fear.[16] [17] [18] Another, hardly less exotic treatment, is burning the underpants of someone of the opposite sex and using the ashes in a way unspecified.[15]

There are numerous reports of koro in non-Chinese subjects, including epidemics which have adorned the pages of *The Lancet, The British Journal of Psychiatry* and other reputable journals. Cases were described in such diverse individuals as a Georgian Jewish immigrant, and a plumber who was born and bred in Bedfordshire.[18] [19]

Obesity

Many biological characteristics are susceptible to measurement. Good examples are height, weight, and the concentrations in blood or serum of many substances. As a general rule these measurements will, in a population, be distributed around a mean in a normal or Gaussian way. This means that most of the values will cluster around the mean but that a smaller number will lie some distance away. This creates a problem when it comes to defining abnormality. Conventionally, values which lie beyond two standard deviations from the mean are regarded as 'abnormal'. This has no logical justification, although it is true to say that the further away from the mean that an observation lies, the more likely it is a true abnormality.

Fatness is one such characteristic. There is no dividing line between normal and abnormal, no clear distinction between health and disease. Nonetheless: 'A National Institute of Health consensus panel on the health implications of obesity has concluded that obesity is a potential killer. It is like blood pressure in that there is no threshold of overweight at which ill effects begin. Any degree of overweight, even 5 or 10 pounds, may be hazardous to health'.[20] This is a quote from a *Science* article with the title 'Obesity Declared a Disease'. The journalist goes on to note that: 'Edward Huth, who is the editor of the *Annals of Internal Medicine*, likened the obesity report to the Surgeon General's report on smoking of about 25 years ago and remarked that he hopes that this report will have the same effect'.

The reality is that the evidence that being a bit fat is bad for you is poor and for minor degrees of fatness non-existent. In fact the plump may live longer than the thin. According to the criteria of the American National Institutes of Health, two-thirds of adult men were obese, that is their weight exceeded by at least 20% their 'desirable' weight. Yet, in several studies, men whose weight was 15-20 pounds higher than their 'desirable' weight lived longer than their thinner peers.[21]

The designation of fatness as a disease has a number of consequences, few of which are desirable. It leads to a belief that telling a person that they are 10 pounds overweight is beneficial, because that will make them weight-conscious. It leads to a belief that taking off 10 pounds will prevent disease and lengthen life. It leads to a belief that it is good for the 'patient' to start looking at food as a source of calories rather than as a source of comfort and enjoyment. This is certainly good for the pockets of those who write about diet and those who operate food-fad stores. Finally it leads to a belief, that by analogy with smoking, overweight people should, even more than at present, be viewed as ugly and irresponsible. Such a belief might lead to the imposition of a 'fat-tax' and the removal of Rubens' canvases from galleries accessible to children. Some cases of anorexia in adolescents may be related to the present obsession with slimness.

Hypertension

Blood pressure, like fatness, is 'normally' distributed in populations, although in rich countries there is usually some skewing to the right; that is, the distribution is not entirely symmetrical and high values are somewhat more common than low ones. There is, as with obesity, a problem in defining what constitutes abnormality and the existence of disease.

Hypertension, high blood pressure, is perhaps the most widespread and damaging of present day non-diseases. The only workable definition of hypertension is 'blood pressure I treat'. A study of the prevalence of 'hypertension' in those aged 50-64 in Australia and the USA concluded that almost 70% of Australians and almost 50% of

Americans were hypertensive: hypertension was defined as a systolic pressure of greater than 140 mm. Hg and/or a diastolic pressure of 90 mm. Hg or more.[22]

There is good evidence that treating the small minority of people who have sustained blood pressure of more than 105 mm Hg diastolic, reduces the subsequent incidence of stroke.[23] Incidentally, high blood pressure of unknown cause, that is most 'cases' of hypertension, is called 'essential hypertension', which sounds much better.

On the other hand the results of the Medical Research Council Trial of treating patients with mild to moderate hypertension (diastolic pressure between 90-109 mm. Hg) with either propranolol or bendrofluazide (a drug which increases the excretion of water and salt) against placebo showed no benefit in reduction of all cause mortality in those who had received active treatment.[24] 17,534 cases underwent 85,572 patient-years of observation. Deaths in the treated group were 248, and in the placebo group 253. Side effects among those receiving bendrofluazide and propranolol included gout, diabetes and impotence.

Those who took placebo tablets did not escape side-effects. By twelve weeks 16% of those men taking the diuretic, 14% of those taking propranolol and 9% of those taking the placebo had become impotent; at two years these figures had risen to 23% in the diuretic group and to 10% in those taking the placebo![25] This suggests that attaching the label 'hypertensive' has, of itself, deleterious effects.

The harm- to- benefit ratio of treating mild or moderate hypertension is, in the present state of our ignorance, adverse; that is, the probability of harm outweighs the possibility of good. The authors of the Medical

Research Council Trial, which is the best, if imperfect, evidence available, concluded that if 850 mildly 'hypertensive' patients are given antihypertensive drugs for a year, about one stroke will be prevented. It is, however, impossible to predict which people are most likely to have a stroke if untreated, 'so this benefit can be achieved only at the expense of involving a substantial percentage of people in adverse reactions to the drugs, mostly but not all minor'.

The likelihood of diagnosing non-hypertension increases with age. Messerli and others found that half of 24 'hypertensive' patients over the age of 65, had 'pseudo-hypertension'.[26] Pseudo-hypertension is an artefact caused by increased resistance to compression of the artery by the sphygmomanometer cuff because of hardening of the arterial wall. The degree of pseudo-hypertension, that is the difference between cuff pressure and true pressure, (as measured by direct intra-arterial measurement), ranged from 10 to 54 mm. Hg with a mean of 16 mm. Hg for both systolic and diastolic pressures. This would suggest that about half the patients over 65 whose mean cuff blood pressure was 180/100, had a true blood pressure of less than 165/85, which is normal for their age and would not justify treatment. If these patients' blood pressure were to be lowered by drugs it would not only be inappropriate and wasteful of resources but would also place these people at the risk of side effects and even of death.

The harms of labelling

When people who feel perfectly well are told that they have a serious and potentially life-threatening disorder, such as 'hypertension', for which they are advised to take daily medication, the consequences are often serious. For example, in a randomised study of steelworkers whose diastolic pressure was greater than 95 mm. Hg, the label 'hypertensive' was associated with increased absenteeism because of 'illness' and decreased psychological well-being: 'The increase in illness absenteeism bears a striking relationship to the employee's awareness of the diagnosis but appears unaffected by the institution of antihypertensive therapy or the degree of success in reducing blood pressure'.[27]

Treated 'hypertensives' are more depressed and complain of more symptoms than untreated 'hypertensives' identified through population screening.[28] Logan remarked on the unfavourable effect the hypertensive label had on psychological well-being, marital life and work attendance. It led to worry and preoccupation with health and to a restriction of social, recreational and occupational activities.[29]

A *Lancet* editorial quoted Milne and others, who observed that both newly labelled and chronic hypertensive people showed differences on many indices of psychological status from controls whose blood-pressure was recorded as 'normal'. The indices included perception of health, total symptom score, worry, and ability to participate in enjoyable activities.[30 31] This did not dissuade the editorialist from calling for a 'vigorous effort to detect the hypertensive subject'.

Psychiatric disease

So far in this chapter we have been primarily concerned with physical disease and have made scant reference to mental illness. For most of us our sense of personal identity and uniqueness lies in our mind, rather than in other parts of our bodies. Losing even major parts - eyes, arms or legs - may dent our self-image but does not threaten our essential selves. Mental illness is a much more personal threat; it is ourselves, rather than some part, that is diseased. Not many people in applying for a job would hesitate to inform prospective employers that they had had their appendices removed, or even that they had had an operation for gallstones, but few would readily admit to a mental hospital admission. If necessary, reference might be made to what is euphemistically described as a 'nervous breakdown'.

The other important difference between mental and physical disease is the difference in diagnostic criteria. The diagnosis of physical disease rests on criteria which for the most part are objective. It rests on signs which can be seen, felt and above all measured; admittedly with a variable margin of error. Yet the criteria which are used for the diagnosis of mental disease are so vague that no objective agreement exists between different schools of psychiatry. Nonetheless the consequences of psychiatric labels are much more sinister.

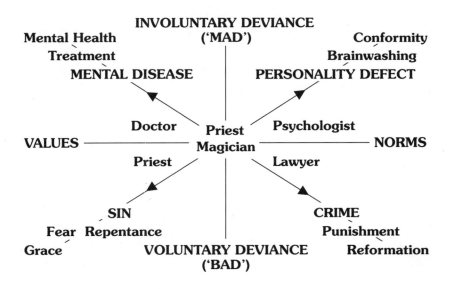

Psychiatric diagnosis

There are certain physical disorders which from time to time abut on the provenance of psychiatrists: such conditions as abnormal behaviour caused by brain tumours, toxic psychoses from drugs, undiagnosed vitamin B12 deficiency, mental handicap and the dementias of advancing years. Yet brain tumours, once diagnosed, become the concern of neurologists and neurosurgeons, poisonings or metabolic disorders are referred to other specialists, and brain failure in the elderly is primarily the responsibility of geriatricians rather than psychiatrists.

For the most part the diagnosis of mental illness is made on the basis of unusual, unacceptable, or 'deviant' behaviour. Unusual sadness is depressive illness; unusual worry, anxiety neurosis; unusual sexual proclivity, perversion; unacceptable minor stealing, kleptomania; excessive or unacceptable use of drugs, alcoholism or addiction. In a sense psychiatry is an accepted method for the control of deviance. This is not to deny the possibility that depression may be due to some, as yet unknown, biological disorder. Many believe that manic-depressive illness is indeed of this kind, but in the present state of our ignorance diagnosis depends upon symptoms and behaviour rather than on any objective test.

In many instances there is doubt as to whether unacceptable behaviours are involuntary, (mad), or voluntary, (bad). It sometimes seems that whether people are incarcerated in hospital or in prison is largely a matter of arbitrary decision. Indeed there are many unfortunates who have had experience of both. Furthermore, some psychiatric labels may carry overtones of moral comment, for example, perversion, psychopathy or sociopathy.

A *Lancet* editorial in 1976 discussed the question 'Is grief an illness?': it concluded: ' ..... the most important reason for regarding grief as an illness is that it would thereby become a legitimate and proper study by medical scientists .... It is over this part of the argument that there is the most opposition from the medical anarchists, who deplore the intrusion of organised medical care as much into what Illich calls natural death, as they do into mental illness and drug addiction'. The editorial then calls for a more liberal supply of tranquillisers to the bereaved.[32]

Seeing God, angels and various fabulous beasts, may be labelled as 'hallucination' by non-believing doctors and as 'vision' by believers. Some eclectic psychiatrists are happy with using both labels, depending on the circumstances. 'Visions' are hallucinations which are considered to be useful to society, while 'hallucinations' are the visions of deluded individuals. 'If you talk to God, you are praying; if God talks to you, you have schizophrenia'.[33]

Psychopathological labelling was described by Ackerknecht in 1943 as a 'modern Ersatz for moral norms and judgement'.[34] Thus various behaviours not approved by the state or not indulged in on a mass scale, are apt to be declared pathological. The transition from moral judgement to medical labelling is insidious in most instances, yet the underlying moral judgement is readily discernible. The abuse of psychiatry in the Soviet Union as a way of controlling dissidence is notorious but not unique.

A lunacy of labels
The classification of disease is in constant flux. New diseases are discovered and old ones dropped. Because there is no need to confirm diagnosis by strict objective criteria, psychiatry is at particular risk of

creating diseases.

Few nowadays would know what drapetomania ('drapeta', a fugitive slave) meant. This disease was rampant among negro slaves in the south of the United States in the last century. The main symptom was an 'irrestrainable propensity to run away'. This behaviour was seen as utterly irrational. 'When driven to labour by the compulsive power of the white man he performs the task assigned to him in a headlong, careless manner, treading down with his feet or cutting with his hoe the plants he is put to cultivate, breaking the tools he works with, and spoiling everything he touches that can be injured by careless handling.'[35]

The use of Latin and Greek helps to reify dubious entities. Agoraphobia, (agora, an assembly or market place), fear of going out; claustrophobia, (claustrum, an enclosed space), fear of being shut in; thanatophobia (thanatos, death), fear of dying. A knowledge of Greek is particularly useful in describing new diseases: silurophobia, fear of cats; kynophobia, common in postmen, fear of dogs; arachnophobia, fear of spiders; iatrophobia, often understandable, fear of doctors; ergophobia, fear of work, or phobophobia, fear of fear. The growth of such useful labels has been hindered by the prevailing ignorance of classics. This is not to suggest that people who become excessively uneasy or agitated in certain situations do not have a real problem; it does not, however, follow that such a problem is a 'disease'.

The British Medical Journal has for some time run what might be seen as an agony column by proxy. In this space, experts respond to difficult problems faced by doctors, sometimes one imagines their own but usually projected onto patients. 'A woman aged 29 has always feared hospitals, doctors and nurses. She does not fear pain, discomfort, investigations, etc. but the power that doctors and nurses have over her. She realises that this fear is unreasonable and yet finds it impossible to overcome. What treatment would you advise?' The expert offers the following consolation: 'This woman's phobia would be best treated with exposure in vivo ... it might be best with this particular patient to undertake, at least initially, weekly therapist- aided sessions...'[36] Afraid of doctors, yet without disease? No, no, iatrophobia demands professional help.

In a recent issue of the *British Journal of Psychiatry* a new disease, 'asneezia', (there should be a better Greek equivalent, e.g. aptarmosis) was described. The disease is characterised by the absence of sneezing or the inability to sneeze. Some 'asneezics' had been cured of their distressing affliction by electroconvulsive therapy! God bless them! The author, delighted by his discovery, calls for a more intensive study of this mysterious disorder, 'since it might throw light on the mechanism of causation of a whole gamut of important psychiatric diseases'.[37] It might; on the other hand it might not!

Gilles de la Tourette, the famous 19th century French neurologist and Charcot's pupil, attempted to put the 'chaos of choreas' in order. He described an entity of his eponymous syndrome, which he considered identical with a Malay condition 'Latah', a Siberian disease 'Miryachit' and with the jumping disease of French-Canadian lumberjacks from the Moosehead Lake region of Maine.

This latter condition, also known as 'the jumping Frenchmen of Maine', has been puzzling psychiatrists ever since and several cases have been described in the American literature. The classic description comes from its discoverer, Dr. George M.Beard: 'I found two of the Jumpers employed about the hotel. With one of them I made the following experiments:

> 1. While sitting in a chair, with a knife in his hand, with which he was about to cut his tobacco, he was struck sharply on the shoulder, and told to 'throw it'. Almost as quick as an explosion of a pistol, he threw the knife and it stuck in a beam opposite .....
> 2. A moment after, while filling his pipe with tobacco, he was again slapped on the shoulder and told to 'throw it'. He threw tobacco and the pipe on the grass, at least a rod away....
> 3. .... I struck him without warning on the shoulder or on the back, or mildly kicked him; and every time he was so struck he moved his shoulders upwards slightly...

Another case in the house, 'a lad of sixteen years of age... jumped when he heard any sound from behind that was sharp and unexpected, and struck and threw when ordered to do so. The crowd around the hotel, partly for my benefit, kept him constantly teased and annoyed, so that when he approached he had a stealthy, suspicious and timid look in his eye, as though he expected each moment to be jumped.' [38]

The Maine 'Jumpers' were celebrated in a local ballad called 'The Jumper'. The hero of this ballad was so badly affected that each time the night train blew its warning blast his wife received a black-eye. It took sixteen black-eyes before his 'disease' led to enforced celibacy.[39]

Miryachit was first described by two American sailors in their account of a Siberian journey. This was spotted by William A. Hammond, the Surgeon-General of the time.[40] The sailors had observed very similar shenanigans to those reported in the Maine lumberjacks. A steward, when suddenly approached by his captain who clapped his hands in front of the steward's face, 'immediately clapped his hands in the same manner, put on an angry look and passed on'. When the sailors asked the captain to explain this apparently strange behaviour, he replied 'Miryachit', which being translated means 'he is just acting the fool'. It is conceivable that ignorance of Russian led to the listing of a new disease in Hammond's 'Index Medicus' under 'miryachit'.

The surgery of labels

The consequences of ludicrous labels are by no means always benign or their harm confined to stigma. In a recent book co-edited by a professor of neurosurgery from Harvard, three neurosurgeons reported on 'transventricular anterior hypothalamotomy in stereotactic treatment of hedonia'.[41] The article was introduced thus: 'Behavioural disturbance manifested by an uncontrollable urge to satisfy personal needs and to gain a pleasant feeling of satisfaction may be called hedonia ... The clinical pictures of hedonia differ according to their social acceptance and classification. They imply not only excessive smoking, tobaccoism, but also excessive inclinations to good eating and drinking, luculianism and bacchism. Some of the hedonic manifestations, such as toxicomania and alcoholism, disturb the existing social order and sometimes endanger it to a considerable extent....'. These authors carried out brain surgery on people who smoked or drank, and in one case of 'nymphomania'.

So far as we are aware, not one word of protest has been heard from neurosurgeons worldwide, some of whom undoubtedly suffer from luculianism, bacchism and other perversions. This is a dangerous road. 'The child who laughs when the Bill of Rights is read will not be stood in a corner and deprived of chewing gum, as now; it will be sent to the operating-table, and the offending convolution, or gland, or tumour or whatever it is will be cut out.'[42]

In 1967, two neurosurgeons and a psychiatrist published a proposal entitled, 'Role of brain disease in riots and urban violence'. The objective was to undertake 'intensive research and clinical studies' of individuals who had been involved; the underlying and implicit assumption being that social disorder had its roots in a brain abnormality which could be corrected by surgery. [43]

In 1973, Paul Lowinger, a psychiatrist, made public a secret project which had been established in the Lafayette Clinic, a university neuropsychiatric research and training institute, following the riots in Detroit in the early seventies. The aim of this project was to subject prisoner-mental patients to experimental amygdalotomies, a form of brain surgery.[44] The neurologist in charge, Ernst Rodin, advocated psychosurgery for 'dumb young males', who tend to become violent when they are treated as 'equals'. Furthermore, as after surgery to the brain, 'the now hopefully placid dullard can inseminate another equally dull young female to produce further dull and aggressive offspring', Rodin thought that they should be castrated as well.[45] Lowinger's intervention and the resultant court case, and other similar cases, led to the establishment of peer-review committees to monitor human experimentation and untested treatments in the United States, and ethical committees this side of the Atlantic.

The need for such controls is apparent when experiments, such as the Tuskegee study of the natural history of untreated syphilis in blacks, could have taken place. This study first involved withholding treatment from 400 poor people who had been infected with the spirochaete of syphilis, and subsequently continuing to monitor their progress for forty years. In return for the subjects' agreement to take part they received $100 and the promise of free burial. This study began in 1932 and continued until 1972 and during this time many papers deriving from the investigators' observations were published in medical journals. It only ended when somebody involved in the study at a relatively unimportant level 'blew the whistle' and made the real nature of the study public knowledge. The study took place under the aegis of the US Public Health Service and the Surgeon-General.[46] Leading medical journals nowadays actively consider the ethical dimensions of work submitted for publication but the need for constant vigilance remains.

The translation game
Enrichment of the medical vocabulary by the addition of a new name is not always synonymous with enrichment of medical knowledge. New terms for diseases may often serve as camouflage for a lack of understanding. A person who comes into the surgery complaining of headache during intercourse, may, or may not, be reassured that he or she suffers from 'coital cephalgia'; that is, headache during intercourse. Similarly a nosebleed becomes an epistaxis, heavy periods a case of menorrhagia, a bruise an ecchymosis, and a lousy head, a case of pediculosis capitis. Fleeting pain in the bottom may become dignified as proctalgia fugax. By pronouncing Greek or Latin, the doctor pretends to be in charge of the daemon of disease. Unfortunately the djinn can seldom be returned to his bottle, as the doctor knows neither the cause nor the treatment of the disease. As Doctor Benway wisely observed in Burroughs' *Naked Lunch*, 'to say treatment is symptomatic means there is none'.

Nostrums for baldness have always had a ready market among middle aged men, whose ego seems to depend upon the density of the hairs on their heads. Now at least one pharmacological firm advertises an expensive treatment to be prescribed by doctors for the dreaded disease of alopecia androgynica, that is male baldness. While it may turn out to be a golden fleece for the company, why should doctors participate in fleecing sad 'patients' by prescribing hair tonic at a cost of £500 a year? To put it baldly, women are smarter than men; rather than waste money on hair restorers they invest in wigs.

Conclusion

Without a diagnostic label the human predicament ceases to be doctor business, hence such labels are a necessary precondition of doctor activity. As doctors are generally uncomfortable about exposing their ignorance, there is a temptation to 'diagnose', to label inappropriately, to create non-diseases. Although attaching dubious labels may be rationalised as a response to patient need, too often the label becomes firmly attached.

Non-diseases have one important characteristic which we have hitherto neglected: they are incurable. Because they are incurable there are no possible advantages of therapy. All therapeutic activity directed at non-diseases is harmful; sometimes the harm is substantial.

4

PREVENTION

The fallacy that prevention is always better than cure
Preoccupation with health seems to be an outstanding feature of the ageing century. This has led to a heightened interest in prevention; in the rich world the focus is on coronary heart disease and cancers but this has become blurred by such vague concepts as positive health and health promotion. 'That living has become so difficult is peculiar, for even the experts manage to die in the simplest of ways' (Erwin Chargaff).

Prevention has a price and sometimes the price may be exorbitant. By staying at home we can avoid death on the roads. While a 'stitch in time saves nine', this may not apply to everyman and every preventive measure. If the 'one stitch' has to be inserted one hundred times to save one individual from the 'nine', it may be unwise to queue for stitching. Similarly the cost of one hundred stitches exceeds by a large amount the cost of nine.

Many sorts of preventive measures depend upon avoidance and while giving up smoking carries the price of pleasure foregone it also carries the benefit of more money in one's pocket. Many other preventive strategies carry prices which are not always quantified and which may be substantial. This applies particularly to screening for disease. This activity, usually regarded as prevention, is nothing of the sort: it is the early diagnosis of disease. The criteria by which a possible screening procedure should be judged have been clearly established by Wilson and Jungner[1], but are often ignored by enthusiasts. They include such things as that the disease should be both common and serious and that an effective treatment is available; other important criteria concern the tests which are used to establish the existence of the disease. If a disease is uncommon in the population being screened, even good tests will throw up a large number of false positives; each of these has to be further investigated and carries a direct cost as well as a substantial burden of unnecessary anxiety and needless, often harmful, procedures. Screening for cancers in general, and breast and cervical cancer in particular, may be contributions to ill health and a wasteful use of resources.

Finally, since death is the inevitable consequence of conception, a morbid preoccupation with its avoidance, and the state of Holy Dread which such fear engenders, may diminish the quality of life.[2]

The fallacy of cheating death
The fallacy of cheating death has been promulgated by the apostles of altered life-style. To those concerned with populations it may be rewarding to transfer mortality from one category to another, but unless such transfer is accompanied by prolongation of useful and happy life it is of no importance.

All living species have a biological life span: plants, fishes, animals and humans. While the upper limit of the human life span may be as much as 116 years, the median, or most usual biological life span, is probably about 85. Some of us may be programmed to die before our seventieth birthday and a few of us are programmed to become centenarians. This programme is coded in our genes and is unalterable, at least for the time being. The old may die with, rather than of, disease.

In the rich world life expectancy at birth is beginning to approach biological life span; so the gains which can be achieved by such presently unrealisable goals as the elimination of cancer are relatively small. It has been calculated that the gain in average life span which would result from the elimination of cancer between the ages of 15 and 65 would be seven months.[3] In Sweden the median age at death from cancer in men is seventy four and for all other causes seventy six; for women the median age at death from cancer is seventy five and from all other causes over eighty. The median age at death from coronary heart disease for men is seventy six and for women eighty two! [4]

Fries, in discussing future changes in life expectancy, anticipated a compression not only of mortality but also of morbidity: that is, we would live to die 'healthy' when our time had run out.[5] Unfortunately, experience suggests that dying 'healthy' without pain is less likely than death protracted by painful degrees. Death by senescence is neither speedy or pleasant. Prolongation of death is not synonymous with prolongation of life.

The language of enthusiasts for prevention is often intemperate. Williams speaks of 'unrealistic expectations that despite not complying with their physician's advice concerning risk factors, obesity, smoking and alcohol, they will somehow escape the penalties of their self-indulgence'.[6] Far from being unrealistic, most do escape the 'penalties', though none escapes death.

The business correspondent of the *Sunday Times* spoke for those who have not been deceived: 'What gets my goat is not so much the raging intolerance of the anti-smoking buffs, hard to take though it is in the light of some of their personal habits, but the outrageous and arrogant intellectual dishonesty of their medical subsection ..... 'Give up smoking and live' .... none of their medical pundits ever bothers to spell out the options. What alternatives can I expect? I suspect that the alternatives are neither markedly more pleasant nor overly long delayed .... What I cannot stand is the bland assumption from the medicos that I am stupid enough to swallow unquestioningly their half-baked arguments'. [7]

Limits imposed by ignorance

Prevention is only likely to be effective when the cause of disease is understood. Since we now understand the causes of almost all infectious and parasitic diseases we are in a position to prevent most of them. We know how to prevent measles and malaria, AIDS and schistosomiasis; that these diseases are not prevented is not the result of ignorance but of a failure to translate knowledge into appropriate action. Because of our understanding we can prevent the ill effects of diets deficient in vitamin C (scurvy), the ill effects of a genetic constitution which prevents babies metabolising phenylalanine (phenylketonuria), and the ill effects of the thyroid gland's failure to produce sufficient thyroid hormone (hypothyroidism). Because of our ignorance, however, we are in a poor position to prevent most cancers and coronary heart disease.

The fallacy of multifactorial aetiology

It is not uncommon for epidemiological data regarding associations to be abused by assuming that an association implies causation. This is particularly likely in the case of diseases of unknown cause. In modern epidemiology, the concept of 'cause' has been replaced by statistical associations with so-called risk factors.

As Stehbens points out, risk factors, such as high levels of cholesterol in the blood, are not causes of coronary heart disease, but associated phenomena such as cough, shortness of breath, or fever in pneumonia. Swamps are not the cause of malaria, and although draining swamps may reduce its local incidence, its eradication can only be achieved by finding the true cause. Confusion between preventive efforts (analogous to draining marshes), and the progress of knowledge (analogous to identifying the Anopheles mosquito as the vector of malarial parasites), 'obscures the clarity, precision and logic of the scientific method, misleading investigators in other disciplines and also the public. It is as unjustifiable as referring to ameliorating factors as curative factors'.[8]

The concept of cause is difficult. Even simple examples, such as being hit on the head by a falling hammer, can be made complex. The immediate cause, that is the falling hammer, is both sufficient and necessary, but the antecedent causes involve being under the scaffolding at the right moment and can be pursued backwards in time to the accident of birth, without which the possibility of being rendered unconscious in this way could not exist.

It has become usual to describe diseases for which there is no known necessary or sufficient cause as multifactorial in origin. This applies particularly to some cancers and coronary heart disease. The notion derives from the knowledge that there are many factors associated with an increased probability of developing disease; nonetheless, the term multifactorial when applied to aetiology is a tautology, which has led to unreal expectations and delusion. All diseases are multifactorial in origin. Infectious disease does not inevitably follow exposure to pathogenic organisms; many other conditions need to be satisfied before disease ensues. Road accidents depend upon the conjunction of many factors: factors as various as blood alcohol, temper and temperament, eyesight and weather. Nobody refers to road accidents as having a multifactorial aetiology; the phrase is reserved for diseases whose aetiology is unknown. The phrase is a synonym for 'unknown' and thus a euphemism for ignorance.

Successful prevention
Preventive measures are most likely to be successful when they do not depend upon individuals modifying their behaviour. The major changes in mortality in the rich world have been achieved by such measures as adequate sewage-disposal schemes, adequate nutrition and better housing. Malaria is best eliminated by ridding the environment of mosquitoes rather than relying on people to sleep under nets or to take prophylactic medication.

Unfortunately most successful prevention depends upon altered behaviour. Even immunisation depends on mothers bringing their babies to doctors and clinics. Not becoming infected with the virus of AIDS depends on a careful choice of partners and using condoms. Not being killed on the roads depends on wearing seat belts and crash helmets, not being drowned upon learning to swim.

Our behaviour derives in the most part from those with whom we choose or are forced to live. If smoking is universal every child will learn to smoke, if alcohol is a necessary part of celebration everyone will drink, if chastity is out of fashion, promiscuity will become the rule. Societal norms change with time but relatively slowly, and not uniformly throughout large societies. It has taken thirty years for smoking to move from being normative, to being deviant, to being sin. Much health education disseminates half-truths and dire warnings, which in the short term have little effect on behaviour. In the longer term the effects may be substantial; the best example is the change in societal attitudes to smoking.

Fear works best when people have recently had a good dose of 'timor mortis', most often a heart attack. The best published results in stopping smoking are in those recently discharged from coronary care units.[9] On the other hand, exploitation of fear in health education may often lead to fatalism. Attempts to frighten the young, for whom death is still a distant prospect, are strikingly unsuccessful and sometimes counterproductive.

Legislation has some effect on behaviour but is seldom introduced until a majority of the electorate has already modified its habits: an example is legislation concerning seat belts. Legislation also assists prevention in relation to such things as food hygiene and water standards.

The major, and utopian, goals of health promotion are the elimination of coronary heart disease and cancer. There are other causes of premature death and disability, such as accidents and some childhood illnesses, which are much more certainly preventable.

Coronary heart disease
Since the Second World War coronary heart disease has become a much more important part of the lives of both doctors and people. It is often

referred to as the modern epidemic, although James Mackenzie saw lots of it as a general practitioner in Burnley at the turn of the century.[10]

Epidemiologists have expressed their interest by examining factors which are *associated* with an increased probability of developing coronary heart disease, so-called risk factors. Risk factors, better called risk markers to emphasise that they are associated with an altered probability of developing disease rather than necessarily being causally related, have been described in numerous prospective and case-control studies. At the moment some three hundred risk factors for coronary heart disease have been described and the list continues to grow. The list now includes: cigarette smoking, high cholesterol, high blood pressure, obesity, diabetes, low levels of high density lipoproteins, high levels of low density lipoproteins, selenium, thiazide diuretics, not drinking, not exercising, not having siestas, not eating fish (especially mackerel), living in Scotland, speaking English as a mother tongue, having a high level of phobic anxiety, being scrupulous about keeping appointments, not taking cod-liver oil, and snoring. The important associations include age, being male, a family history of the disease and - perhaps most important of all, because it is alterable - being poor in the rich world.

Because 'risk factors' are associated with an altered probability of developing disease, it was assumed that an alteration in 'risk factors' would reduce death and morbidity . This led to the belief that identifying 'risk factors' in healthy populations would be a good thing to do. This has turned out to be a dangerous delusion.[11] Dangerous because altering 'risk factors' does little good and may do harm.

The evidence that altering 'risk factors' diminishes coronary heart disease

The best evidence about the effects of altering risk markers comes from controlled trials. In these trials the risk status of half of the population under study is altered by some 'intervention', while the other half continues as before; both populations are followed through time to see whether or not they develop disease. Almost all the studies to date have been concerned with middle-aged men in whom the risk of coronary disease is reasonably high. Such studies are still difficult and expensive because large numbers of subjects need to be recruited and followed for many years.

There have been five major multiple-risk-factor intervention trials, all of which were in middle-aged men. The duration of follow-up was between five and twelve years. [12] The risk factors which were altered by 'intervention' were diet, smoking, and blood pressure; in two studies, attempts were also made to reduce weight and to increase exercise. After 828,000 man-years of study the results were as follows: 1015 coronary heart disease deaths in the intervention groups, 1049 in the control groups; 2909 total deaths in the intervention groups, 2947 deaths in the control groups, a difference of 36: that is, four less deaths in 10,000 men per year. Such a small difference is well within the limits of chance.

Particularly in America the main interest now centres on cholesterol and everybody is being encouraged to know not only their blood pressure but also their cholesterol. There have been three major trials of reducing cholesterol by drugs in middle - aged men whose cholesterol was in the upper ranges of 'normal'. The results after 115,176 man- years of observation were as follows: 92 coronary heart deaths in the intervention

Age-standardised mortality from IHD by county in Finland 1961-87, three year moving averages, males aged 35-64

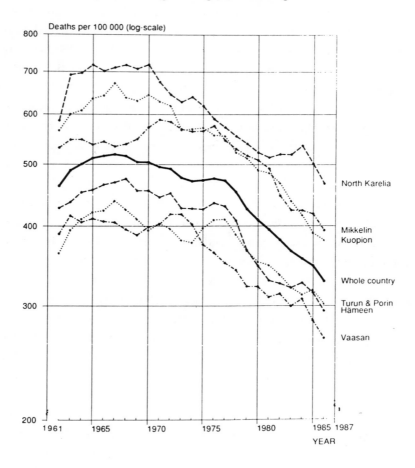

This figure is based on data from the Central Statistical Office of Finland and is reproduced by kind permission of Tapani Valkonen, Department of Sociology, University of Helsinki.

groups, 100 deaths in the control groups; 275 *total* deaths in the intervention groups but only 240 deaths in the control groups. In other words,
lowering cholesterol with drugs did no good and may have done harm.

The other main risk marker is raised blood pressure which we have
already discussed (see page 72). It seems that any benefits which might
result are confined to a reduced incidence of stroke and except for those
rare individuals with very high blood-pressures, lowering blood pressure does not reduce the frequency of coronary heart disease.

Those who advocate the identification of risk markers and who believe
that coronary heart disease is preventable often cite the North Karelia
experiment. North Karelia is a county in Finland, which had the highest
known mortality rates from coronary disease. It was decided that there
should be a major county-wide campaign in North Karelia to reduce
risk markers and that the results would be compared with a neighbour-
ing control county, Kuopio. While mortality fell in North Karelia, it also
fell in Kuopio and in all the other counties of Finland, where there had
been no equivalent attempt to alter risk status.[13]

The other argument which is often used in favour of activism is the fall
in mortality rates which has occurred in the United States and Australia
and some other English speaking countries, and which is ascribed to
healthier life style, dietary changes, less smoking, treatment of blood
pressure and maybe, better management of heart attacks. These data
are based upon what is written on death certificates and a recent careful
study in Minnesota showed no change in the rates of heart attacks
between 1970 and 1980, a time when national rates were said to be
falling.[15] In Sweden, despite a reduction in known 'risk factors', coronary mortality in men aged between 40 and 74 is *increasing* .[14] Another

discordant finding is that in a number of countries mortality rates in men and women are moving in opposite directions. [16]

It has been argued that the failure of trials to demonstrate benefit in middle-aged men is because the interventions came too late in life; this may be so but the lack of evidence should counsel caution.

A more probable reason for the failure to show that this disease is preventable is insufficient knowledge about its cause. The long list of risk markers is a tribute to our ignorance rather than a proof of our knowledge. Coronary disease may not be a single disease; relatively young men's heart attacks may not have the same cause as heart attacks in eighty - year - old women and both may be different from those people who get heart pain on exertion (angina pectoris) but do not suffer heart attacks.

In this circumstance routine health checks which measure blood pressure, weight and cholesterol are more likely to do harm than good. It may be that as a result of future research, probably carried out in the laboratory rather than by epidemiologists, we may be in a position to identify high risk groups, for which there are safe and effective ways of reducing risk and preventing disease. In the meantime activity should be restricted to advising individuals who seek help. It is reasonable to advise stopping smoking, particularly heavy cigarette smoking, and if there is a strong family history of coronary disease early in life, to measure cholesterol and other blood lipids. There is no place for mass screening for risk markers or population interventions to alter the eating habits of the nation.

Screening for cancer

Many people have serious diseases of which they are unaware because they have no symptoms. Screening is the process whereby tests are applied to a symptomless population or group in order to diagnose disease at an early stage. For a screening procedure to be effective the test must be able to distinguish between those who do and those who do not have the disease. In addition there must be an effective and available treatment which will either cure the disease or halt its progression. No test is perfect; all carry a burden of 'false positives', (diagnosing disease when it is absent), and a burden of 'false negatives', (failing to diagnose disease when it is present). But an imperfect test may become acceptable when the benefits of early diagnosis outweigh the harms induced by erroneous results.

The rationale for screening for cancers is based on the assumption that early diagnosis in a presymptomatic stage enhances the probability that the cancer can be cured. This assumption is certainly not universally true; curability depends on the type of tumour and whether or not it metastasises early, that is whether or not it throws off malignant cells which settle in distant parts of the body and establish 'daughter' growths. The nature of the growth is a much more powerful predictor of outcome than the time of diagnosis, whether relatively early or relatively late.

Good tests have high positive and negative predictive value; that is, they answer with confidence the question 'does this person have, or does not have, the disease?' Unfortunately a test's ability to discriminate in this way is also dependent on the prevalence of the target disorder, that is, the proportion of people in those screened who actually have the disease. One of the major problems in screening for cancers is that relatively few people in the population which is to be screened have the disease. Breast cancer is the commonest cancer in women, yet examination of 'healthy' women over the age of fifty yields only two to three cases in every thousand women examined. The frequency of the disease in younger women is much less. Neither 'Pap' smears, nor mammography, nor examining faeces for invisible traces of blood, meet the requirements of good tests. The positive predictive value of these tests is between 1% and 10%, that is, of every 100 'positive' tests, between 90 and 99 are 'false positives'.

Another major problem with screening for cancers is that tests have to be repeated. In the case of screening for cancer of the uterine cervix, recommendations are moving in the direction of beginning screening at younger ages and shortening the interval between screens. This increases the possibility that at some time in a lifetime of being screened a woman will become the victim of a 'false positive' result.

Screening for breast cancer

The theory behind screening for breast cancer may be fatally flawed. This is because by the time the malignant tumour becomes palpable (about 1 cm in diameter), it has been growing for (on average) eight years. Earlier detection by mammography, say two years earlier, can only be valuable if spread of the growth to distant parts of the body is confined to years six to eight. There is no reason to believe that this is commonly the case. Some tumours grow much faster than this and some at much slower rates. Fast-growing tumours are likely to appear as 'interval cancers', that is cancers which are discovered between screening examinations and are therefore 'missed'.

If women with breast cancer are followed up for a long time, it can be shown that they are still dying of metastatic disease thirty years and more after the original diagnosis.[17] Perhaps in most instances breast cancer is incurable at the time of diagnosis and survival is determined by the nature of the growth rather than by the type or time of treatment. Enthusiasm for screening began following the publication of the results of the first trial (the Health Insurance Plan trial), although for many years cancer societies had been stressing the importance of early diagnosis and had been teaching and encouraging breast self-examination.[18] More recently the results of three other trials have been published. The results of all the randomised controlled trials of mammography are summarised in the table below.

Benefit of mammography				
	HIP (New York)	Two-Counties (Sweden)	U.K.	Malmö
Relative risk reduction of dying from breast cancer	35%	29%	14%	5%
Absolute risk reduction of dying from breast cancer	0.02%	0.008%	0.006%	0.001%
How many women would have to be screened for one to benefit?	5061	12, 755	18, 315	67, 568

Perhaps the most surprising finding is that as the techniques of mammography have got better the benefits of screening have become less, and in the two most recent trials the benefit was no longer statistically significant.

If benefit in controlled trials is small or non-existent, what of the harm? The physical harm is of two kinds: overdiagnosis, which leads to unnecessary mastectomy or other procedures, and unnecessary biopsies to prove that lesions detected by mammography are not cancers. In the United Kingdom trial, which took place in Edinburgh and Guildford, 51% more breast cancers were diagnosed (and presumably treated) in the screened than in the control group. Similar 'overdiagnosis' was observed in both the Two-Counties trial (40%) and in the Malmö trial (30%). Rates of mastectomy have increased dramatically in the United States and are much higher than in the United Kingdom, although the incidence and mortality rates in the two countries are little different.[19]

Because modern mammography can detect small abnormalities which have an uncertain nature and prognosis, biopsy rates are increased, and biopsy may lead to mastectomy to be 'on the safe side'. If mammography were universally adopted in the United Kingdom, as has been suggested by the Forrest Committee, we could anticipate something of the order of 100,000 'false positives' every year, resulting in many unnecessary biopsies and an unknown proportion of unnecessary mastectomies.

In addition to physical harm, screening of this kind inevitably leads to psychological harm. For those who have cancer, but who derive no benefit from early diagnosis, screening adds a burden of 'cancer years':

that is, years in which they know that they have the disease and suffer unnecessary anxiety. Undiagnosed, they would have remained symptomless. More serious, because it effects so many more people, is the burden of unnecessary anxiety created by 'false positive' diagnoses. This may well leave wounds to the psyche which will heal much more slowly than the wound of the biopsy.

Mammography is a poor screening test because its positive predictive value in asymptomatic populations is low - between 5% and 10%. This means that only 5-10 'positive' mammograms out of a hundred are truly positive. As screening has to be repeated many times within a lifetime the chances of being the victim of a 'false positive' result are cumulative. The decision of the present government in the United Kingdom to accept the recommendations of the Forrest Report that such screening should be made universally available will, if implemented, do more harm than good. It also brings in its wake other problems which we have not discussed. In particular there is the problem of training people to interpret the large number of mammograms and ensuring that their quality of interpretation remains at a high level. The experience of highly specialised units may not be generalisable throughout a service.

Screening for cancer of the uterine cervix
Cancer of the neck of the womb is much less common than cancer of the breast. Mortality rates are less than a sixth of those from cancer of the breast. It also differs from cancer of the breast in that it is a more curable cancer because it spreads locally rather than by distant metastases.

Enthusiasm for screening began some twenty years ago following the publication of results from British Columbia. The enthusiasm was such as to lead doctors to forecast that this disease would be completely eradicated in the near future. However the findings in British Columbia led others to examine what had been happening to mortality from this disease in other places, including other parts of Canada, where screening was unusual and where there were no organised programmes. They found that mortality rates were declining equally fast in all the other provinces of Canada. Mortality rates were also declining in other countries in which there was no organised screening.[20]

Enthusiasm for this form of screening has continued and has produced a climate in which it has been impossible to mount controlled trials such as those to assess the value of screening for cancer of the breast. As a result, the debate about the value of screening for cervical cancer has had to make do with comparing data from various countries without the advantage of controls for confounding variables.

Screening for this disease is based upon the use of the cervical smear or 'Pap' test, named after Dr George Papanicolau. It depends upon a doctor or nurse taking scrapings or brushings from the cervix with particular reference to the opening of the canal which leads from the vagina to the womb. The scrapings are then transferred to a microscope slide, which is subsequently stained and examined for unusual cells. There are many possibilities for error during this process. The relevant part of the cervix may not be included in the smear, the important cells may not be transferred to the slide, the examination of the slides has to be undertaken by doctors or technicians and they may either miss abnormal cells or describe normal cells as abnormal. For these reasons there is a burden of 'false negatives'.

The other major problem with the test is that although the prevalence of this cancer is low many women's smears show cells which are reported as abnormal and are thought by some to be precursors of malignant change. The significance of these 'abnormalities' is still a matter of uncertainty; it is well established that many of them disappear and yet their existence at least creates anxiety and may lead to colposcopy (a closer examination of the cervix using magnification) and biopsy (removal of a portion of the cervix for microscopic examination) and sometimes to more heroic measures, such as hysterectomy, to be 'on the safe side'. These 'abnormalities' are much more common than the disease and this has led Alwyn Smith, a past President of the Faculty of Community Medicine, to state that 'it is absurd to conduct a screening test in such a way that nearly forty women are referred for an expensive and possibly hazardous procedure for every one who is at risk of developing serious disease'.[21] In England and Wales, according to a *Lancet* editorial, 40,000 smears and 200 excision biopsies were performed for each cervical cancer death thought to be prevented by screening.[22]

If the benefits of this screening test are dubious, the harms are definite. In two recent studies from Britain it was shown that the 'diagnosis' of 'premalignant' disease had significant adverse psychosexual consequences in a large proportion of women. Many were 'devastated' or 'stunned', some lost weight, and some began to brood about the arrangements for their funeral.[23] [24]

The British Medical Journal has a regular column entitled 'Personal View'. A lecturer in medical sociology recently described her experience of having a cervical smear. After her general practitioner rang her to inform her that her smear was 'positive' and that he should make an appointment for a colposcopy, she reacted in this way: 'Surprisingly, given my belief that early detection of cancer carries an excellent prognosis, I reacted badly to the news. For several days I could think of nothing but death'. Following the biopsy she bled heavily (a not uncommon complication) and had to be admitted to hospital, where an inexperienced doctor told her that the blood clot contained a six-week-old- foetus: something which she knew could not conceivably be true. The biopsy wound was cauterised and she underwent a dilatation of the cervical canal and a curettage of her uterus under general anaesthesia. During her hospital stay she was seen by three different gynaecologists, but none gave her what seemed adequate information. Several weeks later she had laser treatment, which was again followed by heavy bleeding. She concluded: 'My complaint is that I was not warned about possible side effects or informed that screening carries its own hazards to mental and physical health. I would still give my consent, but it would have been informed consent'.[25]

The abominable no-men

There is no certainty in science, yet it would be manifestly absurd to allow the absence of certainty to make us eschew action of any kind. All our everyday actions are surrounded by uncertainties. It is difficult to carry out the large scale population studies which would provide good evidence that modification of 'life style' has beneficial effects. This has led to a conflict which is a matter of judgement rather than of fact.

On the one hand there are those who believe that present evidence, imperfect and inadequate as it may be, provides sufficient grounds for advocating changes in behaviour which go far beyond advice on smoking. They would argue that those who counsel caution are delaying the institution of appropriate public health measures, and that by so doing are sentencing many to unnecessary suffering and an early grave. The language of this debate is often more like the language of the hustings than that of academia and those who express doubts have been dubbed 'the abominable no-men'. We are happy to be numbered among them.

Prevention parodies
Traditionally, medicine has dealt with disease, offering the possibility of cure and the assurance of care and concern to the individual who was sick. Recently it has extended its boundaries to a preoccupation with health and is increasingly guilty of offering false promises.

It may be difficult, even for the well informed, to decide what health advice to follow. In order to avoid breast cancer it is wise to become pregnant before the age of twenty; in order to avoid cancer of the cervix, it is wise to remain a virgin. This, however, leads to further problems: childless women are at increased risk of cancer of the colon and of the body of the uterus.

G.S.Myers assembled the composite picture of an individual with a low risk of coronary heart disease. He would be: .... 'an effeminate municipal worker or embalmer completely lacking in physical or mental alertness and without drive, ambition, or competitive spirit; who has never attempted to meet a deadline of any kind; a man with poor appetite, subsisting on fruits and vegetables laced with corn and whale oil, detesting tobacco, spurning ownership of radio, television, or motorcar, with full head of hair but scrawny and unathletic appearance, yet constantly straining his puny muscles by exercise. Low in income, blood pressure, blood sugar, uric acid and cholesterol, he has taken nicotinic acid, pyridoxine, and long term anti-coagulant therapy ever since his prophylactic castration'.[26] Dr Howard has described the person least likely to develop a heart attack as: 'a bicycling, unemployed, hypo-beta-lipoproteinaemic, hypolipaemic, underweight, premeno-pausal, female dwarf living in a crowded room on the island of Crete before 1925 and subsisting on a diet of uncoated cereals, safflower oil and water'.[27] No doubt, in the unlikely event of these two freaks meeting, and mating successfully, their progeny would be doubly blessed.

Prevention as a crusade

These entertaining fancies have a more serious purpose in that they remind us of the ideological simplicity of the quasi-religious crusades against the old enemies, sex, drugs, gluttony and sloth. The false prom-ise of salvation has been exposed by W.H.Carlyon, one time Director of the Health Education Programme of the American Medical Association: 'Constant lifestyle self-scrutiny in search of risk factors, denial of pleas-ure, rejection of the old evil lifestyle and embracing a new rigorous one are followed by periodical reaffirmations of faith at revival meetings of believers .... The zeal with which converts are sought by the recently saved is of awesome intensity ... The self-righteous intolerance of some wellness zealots borders on health fascism. Historically, humans have been at greatest risk while being improved in the best image of their possibilities as seen by somebody else.'[28]

This sentiment has also been expressed by Friedson, an American so-ciologist, who feared that: 'A profession and a society which are so concerned with physical and functional well-being as to sacrifice civil liberty and moral integrity must inevitably press for a 'scientific' envi-ronment similar to that provided for laying hens on progressive chicken farms - hens who produce eggs industriously and have no disease or other cares'. Irving Zola, another sociologist, commenting on this passage, added: 'Nor does it really matter if, instead of the above depressing picture, we were guaranteed six more inches in height, thirty more years of life or drugs to expand our potentialities and potencies; we should still be able to ask, what do six inches matter, in what kind of environment will the thirty additional years be spent, or who will decide what potentialities and potencies will be expanded and what curbed'.[29]

The ethical dimension

Preventive medicine seems to be largely exempt from ethical considerations. This exemption has something to do with the half-truth that prevention is better than cure and the corollary that the self-evident benefit needs no ethical defence. This view ignores the uncomfortable reality that many preventive strategies carry the possibility of doing more harm than good. It also ignores the fact that some present activities are ineffective. There is a temptation to confuse aspiration with achievement.

The exemption from ethical considerations may also have something to do with the historical development of preventive medicine. It grew, in the first place, from the state's interest in protecting its healthy citizens from contagion, which led to the forced segregation of lepers and the quarantine imposed on prospective immigrants to the United States, beneath the Statue of Liberty. Early preventive medicine was synonymous with medical policing. In the 19th century, prostitutes were screened by police surgeons not for the sake of their own health but for the protection of their clients. Screening for disease was initially used as a sieve to separate the healthy and useful from the weak and useless, whether on behalf of insurance companies (to exclude poor risks), armies (to weed out weaklings), or employers (to keep up productivity).

Population interventions which have as their goal the prevention of coronary heart disease and many cancers should be regarded as population experiments and the same guidelines should apply to them as to clinical trials. That many such interventions are of an experimental nature and of uncertain benefit is made clear by the fact that they have been, and still are, tested by means of controlled trials. If a healthy volunteer, or a patient, has the right to be fully informed about the nature of trials and the benefits and risks which might be involved, then even more meticulous attention should be paid to the rights of whole populations of healthy people.

That the position of a doctor offering screening is different from a doctor who is attending to a patient's complaints has been repeatedly stressed in the writings of Thomas McKeown, Archibald Cochrane and Peter Elwood, and David Sackett and Walter Holland - all of them instrumental in establishing epidemiology as a rigorous discipline - but largely ignored by the organisers of mass screening programmes. Cochrane and Holland wrote: 'We believe that there is an ethical difference between everyday medical practice and screening. If a patient asks a medical practitioner for help, the doctor does the best he can. He is not responsible for defects in medical knowledge. If, however, the practitioner initiates screening procedures he is in a very different situation. He should, in our view, have conclusive evidence that screening can alter the natural history of disease in a significant proportion of those screened'.[30]

General practitioners are being exhorted by Royal Colleges and now by the government in the United Kingdom, to become increasingly involved in what has come to be known as opportunistic screening, that is, adding to the ordinary consultation some screening activity such as a blood pressure recording, a cervical smear or an examination of the breasts. Because the benefits of common immunisations outweigh by a substantial margin the possible harms, seeking out children who have not been immunised is ethically defensible, provided that mothers are informed of both expected benefit and possible harm. However, as the benefits of common screening procedures are uncertain and the possibility of harm substantial, there is an inadequate ethical justification for undertaking such tests, unless they have been requested by patients, or they are clinically indicated because of the nature of the patient's symptoms.

It is understandable that a doctor should maintain a certain modicum of therapeutic optimism when caring for the sick, but the extension of this optimism into the domain of preventive medicine cannot be justified; that which provides consolation and a ray of hope to the cancer sufferer may be misinformation or a lie when offered to healthy people.

5

ALTERNATIVE MEDICINE

Throughout history, medicine and magic have been closely linked and, at times, indistinguishable. Pliny thought that magic originally sprang from medicine. Even now the boundary between rational medicine and quackery is fuzzy, partly because medical education does not provide criteria for the demarcation of the absurd.[1] Two things distinguish alternative medicine. The first is that it does not derive from any coherent or established body of evidence. The second, that it is not subjected to rigorous assessment to establish its value. The increasing popularity of 'alternative' healing reflects increasing dissatisfaction with the dehumanising aspects of modern technological medicine and its apparent preoccupation with curing the curable at the expense of caring for the incurable. It is inevitable that those with chronic and incurable diseases and those whose symptoms have been regarded as imaginary, because doctors failed to explain them, will turn for help to unorthodox practitioners.

Regrettably, not all doctors practice rational medicine, and conversely, not all healers are quacks. The effectiveness of therapy is directly proportional to the faith of the therapist and by no means all healers are frauds. However, in the end it matters little whether a healer believes that he acts as a channel for the power of God or that he is an unrecognised Galileo who has discovered 'natural' healing energy or that he sets out to gull the gullible: the means employed are of the same kind. The variety and absurdity of 'alternative' cures is a tribute to the power, largely unrecognised and unacknowledged, of the placebo effect, already described in chapter one. In this chapter we explore some of the techniques of alternative medicine.

The nature of alternative therapies

One reason why the claims made on behalf of these therapies cannot be properly evaluated is the lack of an accurate diagnosis. Some healers, those who are Christian Scientists for example, deny the existence of disease, others do not require a diagnosis, and many have developed their own disease classification, which is meaningless to anybody else: for example, those practising homoeopathy, auricular or 'classical' acupuncture, Voll's electrodermal diagnosis, osteopathy and chiropractic, iridology, Kirlian photography, or medical dowsing.

Alternative therapies can be divided into several categories, which often overlap, and it is not unusual for 'alternative' practitioners to embrace several healing methods in their 'holistic' approach.[2]

1 **Mind cure**: all forms of faith healing, Christian Science, Simonton's cancer cure, psionic medicine.
2 **Medication**: homoeopathy, Bach's flower remedies, herbalism, tissue salts, oral chelation, urine therapy, the apricot-kernel cancer cure, Cousin's and Pauling's vitamin C cure, rejuvenation therapies.
3 **Manipulation**: osteopathy, chiropractic, reflexology, acupuncture, colonic irrigation.
4 **Occultism**: pyramidology, gem therapy, sympathetic magic, psychic surgery, medical dowsing.
5 **Quack devices**: Abram's oscilloclast, ozone generators, negative ionizers, Reich's orgone accumulator, colour-light boxes, black boxes, radionics, electroacupuncture devices.

While many people do not believe in magic as such, they are often prepared to accept magic when it is packaged as science. The anthropologist Hsu recalled how at a Democratic Party Convention in Philadelphia in 1948, many important party members sported Vrilium tubes, which cost $306 each. These pencil-like devices were supposed to emit healing rays which relieved cancer, diabetes, arthritis, sinus trouble and many other ailments.[3] It is a common characteristic of magic devices that they are remarkably unselective and work as panaceas.

In the U.S.A. alone, at least $10 billion is spent annually on what might generally be called quackery, half of it on cancer 'cures'. While not everyone who offers cures is dishonest, a United States committee investigating 'health frauds' concluded that 'incidental evidence accumulated in the process of investigation seems to confirm ...... that many of (the healers) are charlatans'.[4] Even in this case they may be comforted by the rationalisation that their activities have helped people in distress!

Homoeopathy

The examples of alternative medicine which we have so far mentioned are so risible that few of them, although they exist, are important in the British Isles. Homoeopathy is in a different category. It is sponsored by the Royal Family and practised by a number of medical graduates.

This version of sympathetic magic was 'invented' about 1800 by Samuel Hahnemann as a panacea: apart from 'sycosis (fig-warts)' and syphilis, all diseases are caused by a 'miasma of psora (itch)'. Homoeopathists do not treat diseases but symptoms.

The treatment is based on the use of infinitesimally diluted 'remedies', which in higher dose produce the symptoms at which the treatment is directed. Hence the 'homo' in homoeopathy. For example, red pepper gives normal people red cheeks and a feeling of homesickness. A German homoeopath suggested that the 11 million foreign workers in Western Europe would all derive benefit from homoeopathic dilutions of red pepper.[5] The Dean of the Faculty of Homoeopathy in Great Britain prescribes kitchen salt, so diluted that there is unlikely to be a molecule in a hogshead, to help 'a girl with a broken love affair or a woman who has never been able to cry .... to unwind'.[6] This is bound to work, *cum grano salis*, as tears are salty. The same doctor, together with the President of the Faculty, expressed worries that 'ill-trained, un-qualified practitioners can thrive and make wild claims'. Why should anyone need to be trained to prescribe pure water, unless the special training is to facilitate the abandonment of reason and the acceptance of the homoeopathic humbug of 'dynamisation'? 'Dynamisation', or 'po-tentisation' is the process of imparting 'vital force' into the diluent by shaking. The more diluted the solution becomes, if properly shaken, the more potent it becomes and this is why the dilutions are called po-tencies. When the 12th centesimal dilution is reached, known as 12C, the dilution is 10^{-24}. The real meaning of this number is difficult to com-prehend. Perhaps the best way to try is 'Caesar's last breath theorem'. If Caesar's last breath has by now become equally distributed through-out the earth's atmosphere and assuming that the volume of the atmos-phere is about 10^{24} times the capacity of our lungs, then with each breath we take we inhale a single molecule of Caesar's last breath.[7] But 12C is only a beginning; the commonest homoeopathic dilution is 30C, a dilution, sorry, a potency, of 10^{-60}. This is roughly equivalent to one grain of salt dissolved in a volume of diluent which would fill ten thousand billion spheres, each large enough to enclose the whole solar system.[8] According to a W.H.O. publication, potencies of over 100,000C, that is dilutions of $10^{-200,000}$ have been 'successfully' used.[9] That such delusions can capture the fancy of thousands of medically qualified men and women, particularly in France, West Germany and Britain, is an indictment of the education provided in medical schools, or possibly evidence that some minds are congenitally incapable of developing critical faculties.

Numerous trials, carried out when it was still thought that homoeopathy deserved a fair trial, have failed to substantiate its claims. It is difficult to see why there should be a *prima facie* case for such inquiry, and there is certainly nothing to add to the penetrating critiques of Oliver Wendell Holmes, James Young Simpson, (who introduced chloroform), and others.[10] [11] [12]

Yet in the summer of 1988, *Nature*, perhaps the most prestigious of all scientific journals, published an observation from Professor Benveniste, which seemed to materialise the smile of the homoeopathic cat, by claiming, in simple language, that water could 'remember' substances which had once been dissolved in it, but which were no longer present. There was, however, a precondition. Water would only 'remember' if subjected to vigorous shaking between each homoeopathic dilution. Stirring alone was not enough.[13] Other scientists concluded that this explained James Bond's ability to distinguish between Dry Martinis which had been shaken rather than stirred.

Although not mentioned in the published article, this study was sponsored by the homoeopathic industry, which in France is important, as one in four French physicians prescribes homoeopathic remedies. This sensational claim was hailed by homoeopathists everywhere as the final 'scientific' vindication of their cherished beliefs and the media were delighted to report that scientists were 'baffled' by this new discovery.

Perhaps not surprisingly, the editor of *Nature* was attacked for having published 'nonsense' and by so doing giving respectability to such dubious ideas. His defence was that publication and criticism by the scientific community would lay to rest the accusation that the results of homoeopathic experiments were never published in 'orthodox' scientific journals because of pre-existing prejudice; a prejudice which homoeopathists believed arose from the failure of the scientific community to consider it seriously.

Surprisingly the study demonstrated that water samples could have lapses in memory which were not explained by the degree of 'dilution'. (The term 'dilution' is confusing in this context, because frequently not a single molecule of substance remained).

Summer madness reached new heights of frenzy when the editor of *Nature*, accompanied by a professional magician, who had previously exposed Uri Geller's 'psychic powers' as clever conjuring, and a specialist in the detection of scientific fraud, descended upon the French laboratory and asked that the experiments might be repeated in their presence. This request was granted but the original findings were not reproducible in the presence of this team. Within a week another communication appeared in *Nature* , signed by the editor and his companions entitled, 'High-dilution experiments a delusion'.[14]

In the calmer atmosphere of the allergy laboratory of the Rothschild Hospital in Paris, as a result of a request from the consumer health and science magazine *Science et Vie* , further attempts to replicate the water-memory experiments also failed.[15] This effectively ended the matter as far as the scientific community was concerned.

Had Professor Benveniste's experiments been reproducible by others the results for science would have been devastating. The consequences for physics would have been more profound than, say, the discovery that the earth is, after all, flat. Science, as we know it, would have had to be scrapped and rewritten along totally different lines. Professor Benveniste's results were either an artefact of improperly controlled experiment or a miracle, that is a phenomenon which defies physical laws as we understand them. Such earth-shattering observations cannot be based on weak and irreproducible evidence. Extraordinary claims require extraordinary proof.

Dr David Reilly, an eminent defender of 'scientific' homoeopathy, put it well when he wrote immediately after the appearance of the French findings: 'If we prove the observations wrong we will have exposed homoeopathy as one of medical science's greatest misadventures - a folly so massive it will merit study in itself'.[16]

Bach's flower remedies

A variant of homoeopathy, invented by Dr. Edward Bach (1886-1936), was hailed by Dr. Charles K. Elliott, Royal Homoeopath to Her Majesty Queen Elizabeth II, as 'one of the most comprehensive state-of-the-art-systems of healing known'. It rarely happens that a British royal physician, a medicine man of the Bear Tribe in Spokane, and a former New York Commissioner of Mental Health, endorse in one book a panacea - known as Bach's Rescue Remedy. It cures itch, premature ejaculation, the misbehaviour of brain-damaged children, delirium tremens, cuts and bruises, high fever, emotional and physical shock, convulsions and dysmenhorrhoea, to name just a few. It is also useful in the induction of labour. If rubbed behind the ears it revives unconscious animals, and is a wonderful tonic for plants which are 'out of sorts'.[17]

Acupuncture

Acupuncture developed from magico-religious rituals of bloodletting, which were used in China between the third and first centuries B.C. Gradually, pricking at points along imaginary 'meridians' was substituted for bloodletting. The 'meridians' were believed to be linked with inner organs and functions, but follow patterns which totally disregard anatomy and physiology. In its petrified form, this ritual needling survived for 2,000 years, until it was banned by the Emperor in 1822. He removed acupuncture from the curriculum of the Imperial Medical College as a bar to the progress of medicine.[18]

Current interest in acupuncture largely dates from President Nixon's visit to Maoist China in 1970. He and his entourage of journalists and politicians were entertained to a show of 'acupuncture anaesthesia', unaware that this form of anaesthesia was invented on Mao's orders, with the purpose of saving expenditure on anaesthetic equipment and drugs. They were duped into believing that a needle in the ear provided anaesthesia, without realising that the patients, who had been carefully selected and brainwashed, had been given analgesic medication before and during the operation. Similar operations were frequently carried out in the West, using local anaesthesia, but such a normal practice, totally lacking in mystery, was hardly headline news.

The uncritical acceptance of acupuncture was facilitated by certain neurophysiologists who were attracted by Oriental mystique and by the historian, J.Needham, an authority on Chinese science, who endorsed acupuncture as a genuine 'discovery'.[18] On the other hand, Qian, a Chinese theoretical physicist, reasonably asked: if the Chinese had such a marvellous record of scientific achievement why have they contributed so little to the development of modern science?[19] Ackerknecht also pointed out that the wave of interest in acupuncture which followed the Nixon-Mao détente was the fifth to reach the West since the 17th century; the previous waves had all subsided as the true nature of acupuncture as a powerful placebo had been repeatedly recognised.[20]

Because of the interest in acupuncture in such high places as the White House, the National Institutes of Health, universities, other academic institutions and *The Lancet,* acupuncture has become the most thoroughly investigated irrational form of 'alternative' medicine. Numerous controlled trials have shown that acupuncture is no more than a placebo.[18 21] Nonetheless the juggernaut of the acupuncture movement has acquired sufficient momentum to keep it rolling for quite some time to come.

A French acupuncturist invented a new variant, known as auricular acupuncture, which is based on a delusion that all body organs and functions are projected onto the surface of the ear lobe, in such a way that the projection forms a human homunculus (a little man) in the foetal position but standing on its head. The eye of this Paracelsian creature happens to be the point normally pierced for the insertion of earrings. G.T.Lewith, a leading British acupuncturist, was not slow to notice that this might be the reason why pirates wore earrings and that this would explain the old superstition that they were able to see other ships long before they themselves were seen. One of us has analysed the fallacies and fancies of quackupuncture in more detail elsewhere.[18] [23-25]

Needles are needless. The same effect can be obtained by burning cones of dried leaves over the acupuncture points, moxibustion. Or alternatively using a hot iron, or less painfully by applying pressure - acupressure. A special form of acupressure is reflexology: by pressing upon organ projections on the hand or foot diseases can be prevented or cured. For example, in a book on Indian acupressure, prefaced by a former Prime Minister, Morarji Desai, the treatment for syphilis consists of applying pressure over the Achilles' tendon and one ankle while massaging 'the affected part' with boiled urine. In the preface Mr. Desai recommends five other 'natural' panaceas, among them magnetotherapy and drinking one's own urine.[26]

Electroquackupuncture devices

There has been a recent recrudescence of devices which further elaborate and mystify the 'theories' of acupuncture. Two recent additions are Vegatest and the Segmental Electrograph. Vegatest combines acupuncture and homoeopathy. It is an elaborate ohm-meter which measures skin resistance, or impedance, at acupuncture points, in a similar way to a lie detector. The patient is linked to a Wheatstone bridge circuit into which a unit, known as the honeycomb, is incorporated. The honeycomb has a number of holes into which sealed vials of homoeopathic remedies or other materials, used for 'diagnostic' or 'therapeutic' purposes, are placed. The 'diagnosis' or identifying the correct 'treatment' is achieved by reading from a dial which is calibrated in arbitrary units on a scale of 0 to 100.

The segmental electrograph is a more expensive item since it is attached to an Apple computer. It also measures skin resistance, not in one but in eight 'acupoints' at the same time. These eight locations are described as 'quadrants'. The beauty of this test is that it can never be normal: 'There is no such thing as a normal segmental electrogram, as everybody is dealing with many past and present pathological insults of various sorts'.[27]

Both these devices were developed in the 1970's by a German, Helmut Schimmel, and are now being widely advertised and presumably are finding a ready sale. Dr. Lewith and his colleague Dr. Kenyon, from the Centre for the Study of Alternative Therapies in Southampton, now offer courses, not only in acupuncture, homoeopathy and clinical ecology, but also in Vegatest and Segmental Electrography.

In a recent letter to *The Lancet*, the physicist A.T.Barker, who exposed as nonsense electromagnetic healing of fractures, suggested that doctors and the public attracted by unsubstantiated claims for therapeutic and diagnostic properties of various electromagnetic devices should be protected by regulations similar to those covering pharmaceutical preparations.[28] It is sad if such regulations become a necessity.

Osteopathy and chiropractic

A Missouri bone setter, A.Still, had the misfortune to have three of his children die from meningitis. Disillusioned with medicine he developed the bizarre theory that all diseases are caused by pressure on the arteries, mainly in the spine, as a result of structural faults in joints. He discovered osteopathy, as the system is known, in 1876. A few years later, and about one hundred miles away, a grocer and a 'magnetic healer', D.D.Palmer, 'discovered' a competing system, according to which all diseases were caused by pressure on nerves as a result of misalignment or 'subluxation' of the spinal vertebrae. Palmer's first patient was a deaf janitor whose hearing was restored by 'adjustment' of the fourth dorsal vertebra. The mental processes of this Tweedledum of manipulation can be illustrated by a passage from his textbook: 'I am the originator, the Fountain Head of the essential principle that disease is the result of too much or not enough functionating (sic!) .... I have answered the time-worn question, What is Life? Knowing that our physical health and the intellectual progress of Innate (the personified portion of Universal Intelligence) depend upon the proper alignment of the skeletal frame, we feel it our bounden duty to replace any displaced bones so that physical and spiritual health, happiness and the full fruition of earthly life may be fully enjoyed .... I am the Fountain Head of Chiropractic; it originated with me; it was my ingenious brain which discovered its first principles; I was its source; I gave it birth; to me all chiropractors trace their chiropractic lineage.'[29]

Chiropractic, as Palmer's system is known, is advertised as a cure for practically any human illness, including diabetes, heart trouble, tonsillitis or cancer.[30] H.L.Mencken, in his inimitable style, wrote about chiropractic and osteopathy: '(They) counteract the evil works of the so-called science of public hygiene, which now seeks to make morons immortal. If a man being ill of a pus appendix, resorts to a shaved and fumigated longshoreman to have it disposed of, and submits willingly to a treatment involving balancing him on McBurney's point and playing on his vertebrae as on a concertina, then I am willing for one to believe that he is badly wanted in heaven'.[31]

Dr. Barrett described an experiment carried out in Philadelphia in 1976 by the Committee Against Health Fraud: they sent a healthy four-year-old girl for a check-up to five different chiropractors. The first found 'pinched nerves to her stomach and gallbladder', the second noted a 'twisted pelvis', the third worried about future 'headaches, nervousness, equilibrium and digestive problems due to spinal misalignment' which he had detected, the fourth predicted 'bad periods and rough childbirth', if the 'short leg' was not lengthened, and the fifth diagnosed hip and neck misalignment which required instant treatment.[32]

A leaflet published by the recently founded Chiropractic Association of Ireland encourages whole families to come for a check-up 'to ensure early detection of potential nerve interference'. The promised benefits include, 'improved digestion, better circulation, improved mental clarity, normalization of reproductive-hormonal imbalances, and easier breathing'!

The only justification for manipulative techniques are musculo-skeletal disorders, in which massage, other forms of physiotherapy and possibly some specialised manipulative manoeuvres may bring symptomatic relief. However, low backache, which is a common complaint, has a high rate of spontaneous recovery and often runs a fluctuating course, and the value of manipulation, beyond its placebo effect, remains unproven. In a recent trial of osteopathy for low back pain, osteopathy was no better than a placebo.[33]

Miraculous healing

An early form of miraculous healing, which still survives, involved the laying on of hands. Ordinary hands were not considered particularly effective but royal hands were a different matter. *Mal de roi*, scrofula, could only be healed by the touch of a king. The 'royal touch' could also heal many other disorders and it remained a royal prerogative for 700 years.[34] In a delightful account by Aubrey, a certain Evans with a fungous nose dreamt that the King's hand would cure him: 'At the first coming of King Charles II into St. James' Park he kissed the King's hand and rubbed his nose with it; which disturbed the King, but cured him'.[35] The belief is an old one and has its variations. Pliny recorded that King Pyrrhus healed his subjects by laying his toe on them![36] Van Helmont recommended the use of the dead rather than the living: 'try touching the sore with the hand of one who died a slow death, until the patient feels a great chill'; both Robert Boyle, the father of chemistry and brother of the Earl of Cork, and William Harvey tried this cure.[37] [38]

Such notions have not entirely disappeared. A recent contribution published in *The Lancet* said: 'Healing has a long tradition reaching back to Christianity and spiritualism. Some healers believe that their power derives from God, others concentrate on the patient's psychic entity, and others view themselves as a channel through which can flow a natural healing power'. Surprisingly some academic institutions are seriously investigating this possibility.

In Britain, the Confederation of Healing Organisations, which represents over 7,000 healers, are doing their best to have their services recognised as bona fide treatment and therefore reimbursable under the National Health Service.[39] Their president, Dr. Alec Forbes, in a recent article, showed interest in the mystic syllable OM, colour therapy, pyramidology, radionics and homoeopathy.[40] The situation in Britain took a turn for the worse when His Royal Highness Prince Charles became President of the British Medical Association and exhorted the profession to return to the precepts of Paracelsus.[41] Paracelsus' pharmacopoeia included such cures as zebethum occidentale, which was dried human excrement. This could hardly have been beneficial when blown into sore eyes.

In the U.S.A., supernatural healing is sponsored by the White House. President Reagan was among those who congratulated Oral Roberts, the faith healer, on the foundation of his university, the City of Faith.[42]

A British gynaecologist in a recent presidential address confessed that he believed in the miracles recorded by the Venerable Bede and added some of his own.[43] Is there some intrinsic fault in medical education which makes doctors gullible? Sir Arthur Conan Doyle, a medical graduate of Edinburgh University, believed in fairies.[44]

Francis Galton, a distinguished sceptic of the last century, argued that if prayer was as powerful as the religious maintained, it should have some demonstrable effect on longevity. By studying Guy's tables of life expectancy he discovered that in spite of daily prayers for their health and prosperity, members of the royal houses did not do particularly well and, moreover, eminent clerics, despite their apparent life of leisure, had shorter lives than the gentry at large.[45] Galton also noted that missionaries did not live as long as other men, and that churches were as likely to be hit by lightning, set on fire or destroyed by earthquakes as other buildings of similar size. He suggested that the matter could be studied further by examining the relative mortality of babies born to praying and non-praying mothers; a suggestion which might well appeal to present day epidemiologists but which as far as we are aware has not been taken up. A study of the effect of prayer in the London Hospital was carried out but demonstrated no effect.[46]

Believers in supernatural healing tend to ignore the possibility that if good men can heal, by the same token evil men might well be able to do harm. Black magic, voodoo, spellbinding, demoniacal possession, the jinx and the evil eye still plague some societies. In 'advanced' societies black magic has largely disappeared, only the white magic of alternative medicine remains.

Christian Science

According to a senior official of the Church of Christ Scientist, by 'dissolving the mental attitude from which all diseases ultimately stem', hundreds of cures have been achieved in members of their sect. Conditions which have been so cured include cancer, diphtheria, pernicious anaemia, club-foot and spinal meningitis.[47] 'To the Christian Science healer, sickness is a dream from which the patient needs to be awakened. Disease should not appear real to the physician ...... Tumours, ulcers, tubercles, inflammation, pain, deformed joints are waking dream-shadows, dark images of mortal thought, which flee before the light of Truth'.[48]

The founder of Christian Science, Mrs Eddy, discovered her system in 1866. This 'discovery' followed disillusionment with homoeopathy. As, she argued, patients were cured by homoeopathic remedies which contained nothing of their original substance, it must follow that diseases did not exist. Even poisons do not exist in reality but only in the imagination. The reason that people die after swallowing arsenic or strychnine, according to Mrs Eddy, is the false belief that they are poisonous; it is this false belief that is responsible for their death, as arsenic and strychnine of themselves are harmless.[48] The good results of homoeopathy she ascribed to the Divine Mind.

Incredible as it may seem, Christian Science is a recognised 'system of health care' in the United States. The tax-payers are subsidising this form of 'treatment'; the Internal Revenue allows, as tax-deductible medical expenses, fees paid to Christian Science healers. The reason that this is possible is probably due, at least in part, to the magic power of the word 'Christian' and perhaps also of 'Science'.

One doctor has suggested that if Christian Scientists believe that the denial of disease will cure childhood meningitis, as they do, they should also agree to enter children with meningitis into a trial which compared their 'treatment' with appropriate antibiotics, having agreed before-hand that the result of the trial would render the inferior management illegal. He went on to comment: 'neutral readers may be tearing their hair at such a Swiftian proposal, but let me point out that although it might cost the lives of 10 or 15 children (who would die anyway, as their Christian Scientist parents and healers would deny them proper treatment) it might save hundreds from that fate in the long run'.[49]

A coroner in the State of Washington studied mortality patterns among Christian Scientists. On the basis of 1,000 autopsies he concluded that the average age at death was slightly below the national average, and that the incidence of cancer and heart disease among Christian Scientists was higher than the national average.[50]

Mrs Eddy did not adhere too literally to her own doctrine. She consulted a doctor when her husband was ill but even the combined efforts of her healing power and of orthodox medicine did not prevent him dying from an 'illusory' disease. She herself used medicaments, made necessary, as she explained, by the 'animal magnetism' of her enemies.[51]

Mark Twain, the philosopher of common sense, was puzzled as to why Christian Scientists, who claim all diseases to be imaginary, refuse to accept imaginary cheques. 'There is the Mind-Cure, the Faith-Cure, the Prayer-Cure, the Mental-Science Cure, and the Christian Science Cure; and apparently they all do their miracles with the same old powerful instrument - the patient's imagination. Differing names, but no difference in the process. But they do not give the instrument the credit...'[52]

Psychic surgery

In the early 1950's many desperate people went to the Phillipines, having heard of the power of local healers to carry out 'psychic' surgery which not only healed but left no scar. Many of these were people suffering from cancer for whom conventional medicine had little to offer. In the local system of magic, illness is caused by witchcraft: foreign objects, tobacco leaves, pieces of string, broken glass and such like, are introduced into the body by magic and their removal by psychic surgery provides the cure.[53] To conform to the expectations of Western patients, chicken innards and bovine blood provide a more realistic imitation of tumours and diseased organs. The technique depends on being able to palm these objects and to create by their appearance a realistic impression of an operation.

A student of parapsychology, Watson, observed Tony Agpao, whose annual earnings have been estimated at $700,000, remove 'portions of intestine....and a piece of liver' from the abdomen of a woman with 'colongitis' (sic).[54] The patient did not feel a thing and as Watson had provided his own cotton wool there was no possibility of deception! Elementary!?

David Hoy, a professional magician, drew a rather different conclusion: 'as a sleight-of-hand artist myself I was impressed .... in an unguarded moment, one healer distractedly and repeatedly thumb-palmed a cigarette lighter, almost as a reflex action .... In every case I witnessed techniques, moves and uses of suspect props used by professional conjurors.'[53] One such prop is cotton wool: 'cotton wool dipped in oil may be dematerialized into the chest of the patient and a few minutes later rematerialized from the neck minus oil, or it may be dematerialized in one ear and later removed from the other'.[55] This is an old trick which goes back at least to the time of Hippocrates. In the Hippocratic treatise *Epidemics*, a charlatan practice of concealing a wad of wool in the palm and then pretending to remove it from the patient's ear as a cure for earache, is described and deplored.[56]

Driven by curiosity a U.S. surgeon, W.A.Nolen, let himself be operated upon by a Filipino healer in 1973. The healer 'removed' a 'kidney tumour', which looked to Nolen like a piece of chicken fat but he was not allowed to inspect it.[57] James Randi, another professional magician who has devoted much time and energy to the exposure of frauds, was prevented from investigating psychic healing by the Phillipine authorities on the grounds that he might upset 'religious' susceptibilities.[58]

In Brazil, the local psychic surgeon Arigo, was studied by Uri Geller's friend Puharich who thought it significant that during his investigations there was increased U.F.O. activity in the vicinity. According to Puharich, Arigo cured cancer by psychic surgery; in the process he extracted a lot of bloody tissue. Puharich saw Arigo 'thrust' a knife into a patient's eye, without pain or injury.[53]

Some psychic surgeons use 'spiritual' shots snatched from the air which are 'charged' by being placed on the Bible.[53] A Reverend Brown, who seems to have a highly developed sense of humour, snatches a whole panoply of surgical instruments from the air. Equipped with these invisible tools he then adopts an Irish brogue which belongs to an equally invisible Dr. Murphy. It appears that Dr. Murphy heads a team of surgeons, who jointly advise the jolly Reverend which way to 'cut'. The team spirit presumably reassures his patients.

Radiesthesia, radionics, psionic medicine

Radiesthesia, a splendid sounding term, was coined by the dowsing priest, Abbé Mermet. It refers to the ability to pick up 'vibrations' from persons and objects. This groundless notion when used and elaborated upon by doctors is known as psionic medicine. It became fashionable among some British doctors in the thirties, and now they publish their own journal. This science combines the use of the pendulum, homoeopathy and a welter of pseudo-scientific claptrap: for example, all diseases are due to 'over-contraction or over-expansion of the protein as a whole or in many of its parts'.[55] In order to make a diagnosis, the patient's 'witness', which may be blood, urine, saliva, hair, even a photograph or a signature, is set against a diagnostic 'witness', which is an 'inert powder impregnated with the vibrations of various diseases'. Both 'witnesses', together with a homoeopathic remedy, are placed in a triangular configuration and the whole outfit is zeroed with a pendulum.

Radionics uses black boxes decorated with knobs and dials for the quantification of the vibrations; it is high-tech psionic medicine. The first such device was invented by the American medical dowser, Dr. Abrams, who was described after his death in 1924 in the *Journal of the*

American Medical Association as 'the Dean of the 20th century charlatans'. His followers were charged with fraud and some of them jailed. One of them, a chiropractor called D.V.Tansley, came to England, because 'the climate of opinion is a little more tolerant' there. According to Tansley, the patient's problem is sorted out in the box, the 'rate' of his vibration is determined and the 'disease' is cured by broadcasting, telepathically, to the patient. 'Some practitioners will add the appropriate homoeopathic remedy, colour, flower remedy, vitamin or mineral sample by placing it on the treatment set near the blood spot' on the radionic box. For example, a yellow-orange colour is good for liver disease, (presumably because jaundice is yellow-orange), and also for 'hard chronic tumours, idiocy and ulceration of the lung'.[59]

One medically qualified radiesthetist believes that aluminium pots and pans cause 'intestinal toxaemia, heart disease, clots, duodenal ulcer, anaemia and debility.' He determines the extent of the 'aluminium reaction' with a pendulum: if the pendulum reacts to a mentally imagined note, Mi of the Sol-Fa scale after sunset, or to the note Sol during daylight, the aluminium is positive and the patient is treated.[60]

Radiesthetists, together with many homoeopathists, believe that vaccination is bad for health. Its bad effects include growths, hypertension, erysipelas (streptococcal skin infection) and many other skin diseases, including lupus vulgaris (tuberculosis of the skin).[61]

The extensive literature on this subject is characterised, as are many other 'alternative' healing systems, by a medley of fancies: theosophy, astrology, tantric chakras, etheric bodies, and nowadays is likely to be interspersed with references to Einstein, quantum physics and black holes.

Finally, it may be a comfort to note that the presence of a sceptic puts a spanner in the works: 'Experience has shown that should there be scepticism and doubt in the mind of a third party closely associated with the patient .... failure is usually inevitable.'[62]

Conclusion

The claims of systems of alternative medicine all have two things in common. They have no detectable or coherent raison d'être other than the enthusiasm of their advocates and, almost without exception, they claim to cure or alleviate a very large number of ill-defined and quite disparate ills. Some claim to have reached the Holy Grail of the Cure-All.

It may surprise some that we have been prepared to devote so much space to these absurd notions. In defence we can do no better than quote Anthony Garrett. 'On the large scale, history shows that an uncritical and misinformed populace is a breeding ground for all manner of intolerant beliefs and practices. The discovery that truth has to fight for its survival is not a pleasant one, but is an essential realisation in maintaining civilisation. And in a society as open and susceptible to fraud as ours is, truth needs all the help it can get.'[63]

6

MORALITY AND MEDICINE

Medicine and science

'The art and science of medicine' has been the title of many inaugural addresses and valedictory speeches, (a title which is guaranteed to arouse dread in the hearts of those obliged to listen), in which 'art' and 'science', like 'yin' and 'yang', are offered as two sides of the same coin. A coin whose glitter is false gold, as medicine is neither art or science. It is an empirical discipline of diagnostic and therapeutic skills, aided and abetted by technology, that is, by the successful application of science. It is not necessary that doctors should understand the science which underpins their activities. In prescribing antibiotics, detailed scientific understanding of microbiology or biochemistry is not required. Radiological diagnosis does not presuppose a degree in physics, any more than being a competent tailor presupposes a knowledge of the chemistry of polymer fibres.

Science is an activity, not an encyclopaedic body of knowledge. It has been suggested that the scientific method of thought is unnatural.[1] It is certainly unusual; it has to be learned and cultivated. One of the failings of medical education is that, although in the early years there is great emphasis on the acquisition of scientifically based knowledge, relatively few students acquire the method of scientific thought.

Yet without science medicine would still be in the dark ages. Within our professional lifetime there have been a large number of advances in understanding, and consequently in treatment, which have made a major contribution to the quality of our journey from the cradle to the grave; advances which have only been made possible by the work of scientists, most of them not medically qualified, and many working in the laboratory rather than at the bedside.

Ortega y Gasset in *The Mission of the University* remarked that: 'medicine is not a science but a profession, a matter of practice .... it goes to science and takes whatever results of research it considers efficacious, but leaves all the rest. It leaves particularly what is most characteristic of science, the cultivation of the problematic and doubtful'.[2] In a sense, science and medicine are antithetical: science seeks a tentative answer to a general question, medicine seeks a specific answer to a particular patient's problem. The scientist enlarges the pool of common knowledge, the doctor accumulates personal experience. While the scientist looks for new problems and loses interest in them once they have been solved, the doctor who has found a solution is content to become a specialist in its application.

It is fashionable in medicine to pay lip-service to Karl Popper. Presumably if Popper's view of the nature of science is applicable to medicine then medicine, by contamination, is also science. In reality so little in medicine fits the Popperian model of bold conjecture and merciless refutation, that the chief reason for peppering medical writing with references to Popper is rhetorical. Sir Douglas Black, a quondam President of the Royal College of Physicians, in his Rock Carling Monograph, paid the customary homage to Popper, but shuddered at the thought of a 'chaos of hypotheses', which, if Popper were taken too literally, would disturb the comfortable certainties of medicine.[3]

The statement that medicine is not science may well raise doctors' hackles. It is likely to be taken as provocation or insult. Yet an analogous statement that theoretical physics is not science would surely be dismissed by physicists as absurd without a second thought. As a rule, if the epithet 'scientific' is thought to be necessary, the subject to which it refers is not scientific. 'Scientific medicine' is as much scientific as the 'German Democratic Republic' is democratic. 'Scientific communism' is taught in universities behind the Iron Curtain. Acupuncture, homoeopathy, clairvoyance and levitation have from time to time been 'scientifically proven'. None of this worries theoretical physicists; they do not feel obliged to write textbooks of 'scientific theoretical physics'.

The moral dimension
Medicine has a moral content, whereas science is amoral. The neurophysiologist and Nobel Prize winner C. S. Sherrington pointed out that science cannot be bad or good but only false or true. Science is about the pursuit of truth regardless of consequences. The collapse of the dogma which placed the earth at the centre of the universe had earth-shattering consequences for the moral authority of the church, but it strengthened the rational foundation of physics and astronomy. Heresy and science are perfectly compatible.

In similar vein, the French mathematician and philosopher of science Henri Poincaré pointed out that the premises of science are in the indicative mood, and no amount of rhetorical juggling can make conclusions drawn from these premises imperative. The concern of science is about what 'is' and not about what 'ought to be'. Deciding to switch off the life support system is not a scientific question but a moral problem.

Morality and science touch each other but they do not overlap. It is not science which makes scientists immoral. Scientists share moral responsibility with their fellow citizens, and only in this general sense can act immorally. The misuse of scientific discoveries is not the fault of the discoverer, any more than using knives for cutting throats is the responsibility of the cutler. Experiments on human beings or animals, so common in medicine, have, however, a moral dimension. A doctor who, in pursuing his scientific interest, experiments on people without their consent, is practising reprehensible medicine even though the scientific basis of his study may be faultless.

In medicine morality may intrude in both the personal transaction of the consultation and in relation to the public health. It is certainly unreasonable to expect doctors to abjure their personal views, or their notions of right and wrong, good and bad. Furthermore, together with priests, judges and eminent politicians, there is an expectation, not necessarily always met, that they should be above reproach and that their private and personal morality should accord with the conventions of the society in which they live. Yet moral judgements have no place in the consultation, which should respect the individual's right to moral choice and autonomy. This principle has recently been written into the European Code of Medical Ethics of the World Medical Association. Article 3 states: 'A doctor engaging in medical practice must refrain from imposing on a patient his personal philosophical, moral or political opinions'. Beliefs should not distort the interpretation of evidence or the nature of advice. If this does happen, morality may lead to deceit.

Morality and the public health

As Mencken pointed out, 'Hygiene', now known as preventive medicine, 'is the corruption of medicine by morality. It is impossible to find a hygienist who does not debase his theory of the healthful with a theory of the virtuous. This brings it, at the end, into diametrical conflict with medicine proper. The aim of medicine is surely not to make men virtuous; it is to safeguard and rescue them from the consequences of their vices. The true physician does not preach repentance; he offers absolution.' He added: 'We observe quite clearly that the world as it stands is anything but perfect - that injustice exists, and turmoil and tragedy, and bitter suffering of ten thousand kinds - that human life at its best is anything but a grand, sweet song. But instead of ranting absurdly against the fact, or weeping over it maudlinly, or trying to remedy it with inadequate means, we simply put the thought of it out of our minds, just as a wise man puts out the thought that alcohol is probably bad for his liver, or that his wife is a shade too fat. Instead of mulling over it and suffering from it, we seek contentment by pursuing the delights that are so strangely mixed with horrors - by seeking out the soft spots and endeavouring to avoid the hard spots. Such is the intelligent habit of practical and sinful men, and under it lies a sound philosophy.'[4]

Mencken makes the case, more eloquently than we could have aspired to do, for viewing the celebrated World Health Organisation definition of health with suspicion. It does not matter so much that 'a state of complete physical, mental and social well-being' is an unachievable goal (except perhaps at orgasm), although it may serve as an ideal. What matters is that the protagonists of preventive medicine have become the apostles of a false gospel and the good news which they purvey is in the service of a false god.

The present activities of Surgeons General, Health Education Councils and many academic departments of public health and the like, are in danger of corrupting medicine by morality. Smoking has, within our lifetime, moved from being acceptable behaviour, to deviance, disease, sin, and now crime; in Manila one hundred people were recently arrested for smoking in public places and thrown into jail. In the new medical theology, health has succeeded heaven; sanctity is achieved by a 'healthy life style', while the pursuit of pleasure brings the inevitable punishment of disease and death. Rather than admitting our ignorance of the causes of cancer and heart disease and our inability to cure, doctors increasingly blame their patients. Disease is the wages of sin.

Ideas of this kind are by no means new. Socrates, in Plato's *Republic*, expresses horror at the new diseases of civilisation: 'It is disgraceful to need a doctor not only for injury and regular disease, but because by leading the kind of life we have described, luxurious food from Syracuse and Sicily, Corinthian girls and Attic confectionery, we have filled our bodies with gases and discharges, like a stagnant pool, and have driven the medical profession to invent names for our disease, like flatulence and catarrh.'

Foucault, in *The Birth of the Clinic*, showed how, with the fall of religion at the time of the French Revolution, the religious were supplanted by the priests of the body, the therapeutic clergy. The new medical theology created the myth of the total disappearance of disease in a society restored to its original state of health by the unlimited power of a nationalised medical profession to correct, organise and supervise the environment, and to dictate the standards for moral and physical well-being.[5]

The idea that civilisation is damnation and that the 'return to nature' is man's salvation expresses mankind's yearning for the lost paradise, that never was. Tissot, a French medical authority of the 18th century, believed that 'before the advent of civilisation, people had only the simplest, most necessary diseases. Peasants and workers remain close to the basic nosological rule; the simplicity of their lives allows it to show through in its reasonable order; they have none of those variable, complex, intermingled nervous ills, but down-to-earth apoplexia, or uncomplicated attacks of mania. As one improves one's condition of life, and as the social network tightens its grip around individuals, health seems to diminish by degrees, diseases become diversified, and combine with one another; their number is already great in the superior order of the bourgeois.'[6] Such childlike naiveté, attractive to many because of its very simplicity, characterises much of today's health promotion, which would have us believe that the major 'diseases of civilisation' are preventable, if only the citizens were to follow the path of righteousness.

Eugène Delacroix, perhaps influenced by contemporary propaganda, wrote in his diary that by increasing luxury many 'have fatally affected the health of generations to come and have brought about a general decline in morals. We borrow from nature such poisons as tobacco and opium and use them as instruments of our gross pleasures, and we are punished by loss of energy and the degradation of our minds. Entire nations have been reduced to a form of slavery by immoderate use of stimulants and strong drink. No sooner do nations reach a certain stage of civilisation than they find themselves growing weaker, especially in their standards of courage and morality. This general loss of energy, which is probably the result of increase in pleasure and easy living, brings them to swift degeneration and to the neglect of the tradition that was their safeguard - their standard of national honour'.

Concern for 'national health' is one of the hallmarks of totalitarian societies and is usually about fitness to work and fitness to fight rather than individual well-being. The Turkish Sultan Murad IV made smoking a capital offence because he believed that tobacco reduced the fertility of his subjects and the fighting quality of his soldiers.[7] In his *Counterblast to Tobacco*, James I worried that smoking, apart from being a Godless waste, disables subjects 'who are created and ordained by God to bestowe both persons and goods for the maintenance of the honor and safetie of King and Commonwealth.' Compare this with Hitler's observation: 'I am convinced that if I had been a smoker I would never have been able to bear the cares and anxieties which have been a burden to me for so long. Perhaps the German people owes its salvation to the fact.'[8]

7

ENVOI

A book which bears as its title 'Follies and Fallacies in Medicine' can hardly be expected to extol medicine's achievements. The collection which we have compiled may give the false impression that doctors are at best charlatans and at worst rogues, and that medicine is itself a major threat to health. Medicine only becomes a threat to health if it remains untempered by the use of rational inquiry and criticism. Such criticism is an important and relatively neglected task.

Because of its social function, medicine relies on authority and dogma, and those who threaten its beliefs are likely to be branded as nihilists, iconoclasts, or worse. 'Iconoclast', as defined by Ambrose Bierce, is 'a breaker of idols, the worshippers whereof are imperfectly gratified by the performance, and most strenuously protest that he unbuildeth but does not reedify, that he pulleth down but pileth not up. For the poor things would have other idols in place of those he thwacketh upon the mazzard and dispelleth. But the iconoclast saith: 'Ye shall have none at all, for ye need them not; and if the rebuilder fooleth round hereabout, behold I will depress the head of him and sit thereon till he squawk it.'[1]

The reaction of the medical profession to criticism sometimes seems to have an almost paranoid quality. Dollery speaks of 'a paradox that serious criticism of scientific medicine has arisen when its achievements are at a peak and show no signs of decline.'[2] Such sentiments are by no means novel. They were abroad in the middle of the last century: 'at no period have the means for the acquirement or diffusion of medical knowledge been more various and multiplied than the present ... and yet, strange to say, the esteem and respect in which the medical profession is held by the better informed members of society and the public at large was never at a lower ebb than at this time.'[3]

This is not the place to enumerate all the major advances of medicine since the turn of the century. Death around the time of birth and in infancy has become a rarity. Life expectancy at birth has dramatically increased and for many the quality of life has been enhanced. Nobody needs to die from vitamin deficiency. Most infectious diseases are now preventable, and few now die of infection unless they are especially vulnerable on account of age, disease or drugs. Treatment of endocrine disorders, such as diseases of the thyroid gland and diabetes, has been revolutionised by better understanding. New drugs have simplified and made much more effective the treatment of such common conditions as duodenal ulcer and heart failure. Surgery can, thanks to advances in anaesthesia and surgical technique, restore sight to those blind as a result of cataracts, painless walking to those with arthritic hips, hearing to some of the deaf and full health to some of the victims of violence on the roads. The fact that these achievements have had little or no bearing on the lives of all those millions of our fellows which are still 'nasty, poor, brutish, solitary and short'[4] is an indictment of our selfish world.

This book does not aspire to provide simple solutions to complex problems. It is no more than a contribution to the limitation of error. Scepticism is the scalpel which frees accessible truth from the dead tissue of unfounded belief and wishful thinking. The demarcation of ignorance and the exposure of folly may diminish harm, and by removing some of the rubble which impedes the way forward, accelerate progress.

CHAPTER 1

1. The Placebo in medicine: Editorial. Medical Press, June 18, 1890, p. 642.

2. Platt R : Two essays on the practice of medicine. Lancet 1947; ii: 305-307.

3. Maimon KL, Morelli HF : Clinical Pharmacology. Basic Principles in Therapeutics. Second Edition. Macmillan, New York, 1978.

4. Thomas KB : General practice consultations: is there any point in being positive? Br Med J 1987; 294: 1200-1202.

5. Asher R : Talking Sense. Jones FA, Ed. Pitman Medical, London 1972, p.47.

6. Shall I please? Editorial. Lancet 1983; ii: 1465-1466.

7. See 5.

8. Pepper OHP. A note on placebo. Trans Stud Coll Physcns Phil. 1945; 13: 81-84.

9. Montaigne M. Essais I, xxi (De la force de l'imagination). 1580

10. Hippocrates, vol ii. Jones WHS, Tr. and Ed., W. Heinemann, London,1923, p.203.

11. Theophrastus, Enquiry into Plants. Tr. Sir Arthur Holt. W. Heinemann, London,1916, p.313.

12. Helman CG : Feed a cold and starve a fever - folk models of infection in an English suburban community and their relation to medical treatment. Culture, Medicine and Psychiatry 1978; 2: 107-137.

13. Blackwell B, Bloomfield SS, Buncher CR : Demonstration to medical students of placebo response and non-drug factors. Lancet 1972; i: 1279-1282.

14. Black D : An Anthology of False Antitheses. Rock Carling Monograph. Nuffield Provincial Hospitals Trust, London,1984.

15. Gowdey CW, Hamilton JT, Philp RB: A controlled clinical trial using placebos in normal subjects: a teaching exercise. Canad Med Assoc J 1967; 96: 1317-1322

16. Pickering G : Therapeutics. Art or science? JAMA 1979; 242: 649-653.

17. Chalmers I : Scientific inquiry and authoritarianism in perinatal care and education. Birth 1983; 10: 151-166.

18. See 14.

19. Blau JN: Clinician and placebo. Lancet 1985; i: 344.

20. Cobb LA, Thomas GI, Dillard DH, Merindino KA, Bruce RA : An evaluation of internal-mammary artery ligation by a double-blind technic. New Engl J Med 1959; 260: 1115-1118.

21. Diamond EG, Kittle CF, Crockett JE : Comparison of internal mammary artery ligation and sham operation for angina pectoris. Am J Cardiol 1960; 5: 484-486.

22. Beecher HK : Surgery as placebo. JAMA 1961; 176: 1102-1107.

23. Lowinger P, Dobie S : A study of placebo response rates. Arch Gen Psychiat 1969; 20: 84-88.

24. Gracely RH, Dubner R, Deeter WR, Wolskee PJ : Clinicians' expectations influence placebo analgesia. Lancet 1985; i: 43.

25. Sebeok TA, Rosenthal R, Eds : The Clever Hans Phenomenon: Communications with horses, whales, apes and people. Ann N Y Acad Sci Vol 364, New York Academy of Science, 1981.

26. Byington RP, Curb JD, Mattson ME : Assessment of double-blindness at the conclusion of the beta-blocker heart attack trial. JAMA 1985; 253: 1733-1736.

27. Wolf S : Effects of suggestions and conditioning on the action of chemical agents in human subjects - the pharmacology of placebo. J Clin Invest 1950; 29: 100-109.

28. Lindahl O, Lindwall L : Is all therapy just a placebo effect? Metamedicine 1982; 3: 255-259.

29. Spiro HM : Doctors, Patients, and Placebos. Yale Univ. Press, New Haven, 1986.

30. Goodwin JS, Goodwin JM, Vogel AV : Knowledge of the use of placebos by house officers and nurses. Ann Intern Med 1979; 91: 106-110.

31. Lasagna L, Mosteller F, von Felsinger JM, Beecher HK : A study of the placebo response. Am J Med 1954; 16: 770-779.

32. Skrabanek P : Acupuncture: past, present and future. In: Stalker D, Glymour C, eds. Examining Holistic Medicine. Prometheus Press, Buffalo, 1985,pp. 181-196.

CHAPTER 2

1.   Broad W, Wade N : The Betrayers of Truth. Century Publishing, London, 1982.

2.   Krohn A : False Prophets. Blackwell, London, 1986.

3.   Rotkin ID : Sexual characteristics of a cervical cancer population. Am J Public Health 1967; 57: 815-829.

4.   Gibbons RD, Davis JM : The price of beer and the salaries of priests: analysis and display of longitudinal psychiatric data. Arch Gen Psychiat 1984; 41: 1183-94.

5.   Weller MPI, Weller B : Crime and psychopathology. Br Med J 1986; 292: 55-56.

6.   Robinson AA : The prediction of lung cancer in Australia 1939-1981. Med Hypotheses. 1986; 21: 409-419.

7.   The anomaly that wouldn't go away. Editorial. Lancet. 1978; ii: 978.

8.   Wessex Positive Health Team : Promoting the use of seat belts. Br Med J 1980; 281: 1477-1478.

9.   Sterling TD : Filtering information about occupation, smoking and disease. J Chron Dis 1984; 37: 227-230.

10.   Waldron HA : Hippocrates and lead. Lancet 1973; ii: 626.

11.   Hamblin TJ : Fake! Br Med J 1981; 283: 1671.

12.   Aubrey J : Brief Lives. D L Dick, Ed.
      Secker and Warburg, London,1958, p.128.

13.   Fifield D : Nature, 1869-1969. New Scientist 1969; 44 (No.673): 230-232.

14. Yallow RS : Radioimmunoassay: A probe for the fine structure of biological systems. Science 1978; 200: 1236-1245.

15. Thorup OA : Jefferson's admonition.
    Mayo Clin Proc 1972; 47: 199-201

16. Whitla W : Sir Isaac Newton's Daniel and the Apocalypse. With an introductory study of the nature and cause of unbelief, or miracles and prophecy. J Murray, London, 1922.

17. Another Berlin'Cure' for Consumption. Editorial. Medical Press Dec 5 1900, p.604.

18. Moertel CG, Fleming TR, Creagan ET et al. : High dose vitamin C versus placebo in the treatment of patients with advanced cancer who had no prior chemotherapy. A randomized controlled trial. New Engl J Med 1985; 312: 134-141.

19. Derby BM, Ward JW : The myth of red urine due to phenytoin. JAMA 1983; 249: 1723-1724.

20. Cohen L, Rothschild H : The bandwagons of medicine.
    Persp Biol Med 1979; 22: 531-538.

21. Sackett DL, Haynes RB, Tugwell P : Clinical Epidemiology. A Basic Science for Clinical Medicine. Little Brown & Co., Boston/Toronto, 1985, p.226.

22. Skrabanek P : Haemodialysis in schizophrenia : déjà vu or ideé fixe. Lancet 1982; i: 1404-1405.

23. Wiener AS : Blood groups and disease. A critical review. Lancet 1962; i: 813-816.

24. An ulcer in the family. Editorial. Br Med J 1976; 3: 444.

25. O'Connell DL, Hulka BS, Chambless LE, Wilkinson WE, Deubner DC : Cigarette smoking, alcohol consumption, and breast cancer risk. J Natl Cancer Inst 1987; 78: 229-234.

26. WHO collaborative study of neoplasia and steroid contraceptives. Invasive cervical cancer and combined oral contraceptives. Br Med J 1985; 290: 961

27. Fortney JA, Potts M, Bonhomme M : Invasive cancer and combined oral contraceptives. Br Med J 1985; 290: 1587.

28. Hickey RJ : Risks associated with exposure to radiation: science, pseudoscience, and opinion. Health Physics 1985; 49: 949-952.

29. Mather HG, Pearson NG, Read KLQ, et al. : Acute myocardial infarction: home and hospital treatment. Br Med J 1971; iii: 925-929.

30. Mather HG, Morgan DC, Pearson NG, et al. : Myocardial infarction: a comparison between home and hospital care for patients. Br Med J 1976; i: 925-9.

31. Hill JD, Hampton JR, Mitchell JRA : A randomised controlled trial of home-vs-hospital management for patients with suspected myocardial infarction. Lancet 1978; i : 837-41.

32. Chalmers I : Scientific inquiry and authoritarianism in perinatal care and education. Birth 1983; 10: 151-166.

33. Hill AB : Personal view. Br Med J 1985; 290: 1074.

34. Medawar P : A bouquet of fallacies from medicine and medical science with a sideways glance at mathematics and logic. In: Lying truths, Duncan R, Weston-Smith M, Eds., Pergamon,

Oxford, 1979, pp. 98-105.

35. Mencken HL : Prejudices. 6th Series. Jonathan Cape, London, 1928, p.237.

36. Bailar JC : Science, statistics and deception. Ann Intern Med 1986; 104: 259-260.

37. Shapiro S : The decision to publish: ethical dilemmas. J Chron Dis 1985; 38: 365-372.

38. Mantel N : Cautions on the use of medical databases. Statistics in Medicine 1983; 2: 355-362.

39. Feinstein AR : The intellectual crisis in clinical medicine: medaled models and muddled science. Persp Biol Med 197; 30: 215-230.

40. Medical and Physical Journal 1812; 27 (No.155): 8.

41. Lancet 1975; ii: 824.

42. Asher R : Medicine and meaning. Lancet 1943; i: 213-214.

43. Houston CS, Swischuk LE : Varus and valgus - no wonder they are confused. New Engl J Med 1980; 302: 471-472.

44. Chatel J C, Peele R : A centennial review of neurasthenia. Am J Psychiat 1970; 1404-1413.

45. Martin B : Bias of Science. Society for Social Responsibility in Science. Canberra, Australia, 1979.

46. Russell B : Sceptical Essays. Allen and Unwin, London, 1928.

47. Lyttleton RA : The Gold Effect. In: Lying Truths. A critical scrutiny of current beliefs and conventions. Duncan R, Weston-Smith M, Eds. Pergamon Press, Oxford, 1979, pp. 182-198.

48. Hilfiker D : Facing our mistakes. New Engl J Med 1984; 310: 118-122.

49. McIntyre N, Popper K : The critical attitude in medicine. Br Med J 1983; 287: 1919-1923.

50. Featherstone HJ, Beitman BD, Irby DM : Distorted learning from unusual anecdotes. Med Education 1984; 18: 155-158.

51. Maher JP : The dethroning of Thomas Crapper. In: The How, Why, and Whence of Names. Callay E, Seits L Eds. De Kalb: Illinois Name Society, 1984, pp. 123-124.

CHAPTER 3

1. Sackett DL, Haynes RB, Tugwell P : Clinical Epidemiology. Little Brown, Boston, 1985.

2. McWhinney IR : An Introduction to Family Medicine. Oxford Univ. Press, London, 1981.

3. Elstein AS, Shulman LS, Sprafka SH : Medical Problem Solving. Harvard Univ. Press, Cambridge, Mass., 1978.

4. Macartney FJ : Diagnostic logic. Br Med J 1987; 295: 1325-1331.

5. McCormick JS : Diagnosis: the need for demystification. Lancet 1986; ii:1434-1435.

6. Thomas KB : The consultation and the therapeutical illusion. Br Med J 1978; i: 1327-1328.

7. Thomas KB: General practice consultations: is there any point in being positive? Br Med J 1987; 294: 1200-1202.

8. Scheff TU : Decision rules, types of error, and their consequences in medical diagnosis. In: Basic Readings in Medical Sociology. Tuckett D, Kaufert J M, Eds. Tavistock Publications, London, 1978. (Reprinted from: Behavioural Science 1963; 8: 97-107).

9. Meador CK : The art and science of non-disease. New Engl J Med 1965; 272: 92-95.

10. Hart FD : The importance of non-disease. Practitioner 1973; 211: 193-196.

11. Garland : 1969, quoted by Scheff, see 6.

12. Gross F : The emperor's clothes syndrome. New Engl J Med 1971; 285: 863.

13. Weinstein RA, Stamm WE : Pseudoepidemics in hospital. Lancet 1977; ii : 862-864.

14. Impact of swine non-flu. Editorial. Lancet 1982; ii: 1029.

15. Gwee AL : Koro: its origin and nature as a disease entity. Singapore Med J 1968; 9: 3-6.

16. Chong Tung Mun : Epidemic koro in Singapore. Br Med J 1968; i: 640.

17. Gwee AL : Koro - a cultural disease. Singapore Med J 1963; 4: 119-122.

18. Hes JP, Nassi G : Koro in a Yemenite and a Georgian Jewish immigrant. Confinia Psychiatrica 1977; 20: 180-184.

19. Berrios GE, Morley SJ : Koro-like symptom in a non-Chinese subject. Br J Psychiat 1984; 145: 331-334.

20. Kolata G : Obesity declared a disease. Science 1985; 227: 1019-1020.

21. Gordon T, Doyle ST : Weight and mortality in men: the Albany study. Int J Epidemiol 1988; 17: 77-81.

22. MacMahon SW, Leeder SR : Blood pressure levels and mortality from cerebrovascular disease in Australia and the United States. Am J Epidemiol 1984; 120: 865-875.

23. Veterans Administration Co-operative Study Group : Effects of treatment on morbidity in hypertension II. Results in patients with diastolic pressure averaging 90 through 114 mm Hg.

JAMA 1970; 213: 1143-1152.

24. Medical Research Council Working Party : MRC trial of treatment of mild hypertension: principal results.
Br Med J 1985; 291: 97-104.

25. Medical Research Council Working Party : Adverse reactions to bendrofluazide and propranolol. Lancet 1981; ii: 632.

26. Messerli FH, Ventura HO, Amodeo C : Osler's maneuver and pseudo-hypertension. New Engl J Med 1985; 312: 1548-1551.

27. Haynes RB, Sackett DL, Taylor DW, Gibson ES, Johnson AL : Increased absenteeism from work after detection and labelling of hypertensive patients. New Engl J Med 1978; 299: 741-744.

28. Steptoe A, Melville D : Mental health and hypertension. Lancet 1984; ii: 457-458.

29. Logan AG : Mental health and hypertension. Lancet 1984; ii: 597.

30. More on hypertension labelling : Editorial.
Lancet 1985; i: 1138-1139.

31. Milne BJ, Logan AG, Flanagan PT : Alteration in health perception and life-style in treated hypertensives.
J Chronic Dis 1985; 38: 37- 45.

32. Is grief an illness? : Editorial. Lancet 1976; ii: 134.

33. Szasz T : The Second Sin. Doubleday, New York, 1973, p. 101.

34. Ackerknecht EH : Psychopathology, primitive medicine and primitive culture. Bull Hist Med 1943; 14: 30-67.

35. Dysaesthesia aethiopica : Editorial.
Medical Times & Gazette 1856; 34: 472-473.

36. Br Med J 1986; 293: 26.

37. Shukla GD : Asneezia - a hitherto unrecognized psychiatric symptom. Br J Psychiat 1985; 147: 564-565.

38. Beard GM : Experiments with the 'jumpers' of Maine. Popular Science Monthly 1880; 18: 170-173.

39. Kunkle EC : The 'jumpers' of Maine. Past history and present status. J Maine Med Assoc 1965; 56: 191-193.

40. Hammond WA : Miryachit, a newly described disease of the nervous system. N Y Med J 1884; 39: 191-192.

41. Sweet WH, Obrador S, Martin-Rodriquez JG Eds. Neurological treatment in psychiatry, pain, and epilepsy. University Park Press, Baltimore, 1977.

42. Mencken HL : Prejudices. Sixth Series, J. Cape, London 1928.

43. Erwin F, Mark V, Sweet W : Role of brain disease in riots and urban violence. JAMA 1967; 201: 895.

44. Lowinger P : Two comments on psychosurgery. New Engl J Med 1987; 316: 114

45. Breggin PR : Psychosurgery for political purposes. The Duquesne Law Review 1975; 13: 841-862.

46. Jones JH : Bad Blood: the Tuskegee Syphilis Experiment. The Free Press, New York, 1981.

CHAPTER 4

1.   Wilson JMG, Jungner G : Principles and practice of screening for disease. Public Health Papers no 34. WHO, Geneva, 1968.

2.   McCormick JS, Skrabanek P : Holy dread.
     Lancet 1984; ii: 1455-1456.

3.   Tsai Sp, Lee ES, Hardy RJ : The effect of a reduction in leading causes of death: potential gains in life expectancy.
     Am J Publ Health 1978; 68: 966-971

4.   Jannerfeldt E, Horte L-G : Median age at death as an indicator of premature mortality. Br Med J 1988; 296: 678-681.

5.   Fries JF : Aging, natural death, and the compression of morbidity.
     New Engl J Med 1980; 303: 130-135.

6.   Williams PA : A productive history and physical examination in the prevention and early detection of cancer.
     Cancer 1981; 47: 1146-50.

7.   Walker F : Pleasures of smoking: in the end we are all dead anyway. Sunday Times, Feb 17th, 1980.

8.   Stehbens WE : The concept of cause in disease.
     J Chron Dis 1985; 38: 947-950.

9.   Hickey N, Graham I, Kennedy C et al : Trends in response to antismoking advice in patients with coronary heart disease between 1961 and 1975. Irish J Med Sci 1981; 150: 262-264.

10. McCormick JS : James Mackenzie and coronary heart disease.
     J Roy Coll Gen Pract 1981; 31: 26.

11. McCormick JS : The multifactorial aetiology of coronary heart disease: a dangerous delusion. Persp Biol Med 1988; 32: 103-108.

12. McCormick JS, Skrabanek P : Coronary heart disease is not preventable by population interventions. Lancet 1988; ii: 839-841.

13. Salonen JT, Puska P, Mustaniemi H : Changes in morbidity and mortality during comprehensive five-year community programme to control cardiovascular diseases during 1972-7 in North Karelia. Br Med J 1979; ii: 1178-83.

14. Alfredsson L, Ahlbom A : Increasing incidence and mortality from myocardial infarction in Stockholm county. Br Med J 1983; 286: 1931-1933.

15. Burke GL, Edlavitch SA, Crow RS : The effects of diagnostic criteria on trends in coronary heart disease morbidity: the Minnesota heart survey. J Clin Epidemiol 1989; 42: 17-24.

16. Thom TJ, Epstein FH, Feldman JJ, Leaverton PE : Trends in total mortality and mortality from heart disease in 26 countries from 1950 to 1978. Int J Epidemiol 1985;14: 510-520.

17. Hibberd AD : Surgery - prolonged survival or cure? In: Breast Cancer. Treatment and Prognosis. B. Stoll, Ed. Blackwell, Oxford, 1986, pp. 3-12.

18. Hoffman FL: The Mortality from Cancer throughout the World. Prudential Press, Newark NJ, 1915.

19. Greenberg ER, Stevens M : Recent trends in breast surgery in the United States and the United Kingdom Br Med J 1986; 292: 1487-1491.

20. Skrabanek P : Cervical cancer screening : the time for reappraisal. Canad J Public Health 1988; 79: 86-89.

21. Smith A : Cervical cytology screening. Br Med J 1988; 296: 1670.

22. Cancer of the cervix - death by incompetence. Editorial. Lancet 1985; ii : 363-364.

23. Campion MJ, Brown JR, McCance DJ, et al : Psychosexual trauma of an abnormal cervical smear. Br J Obstet Gynaecol 1988: 95; 175-181.

24. Posner T, Vessey M : Prevention of Cervical Cancer. The Patient's View. King's Fund Publishing Office, London, 1988.

25. Britten N : Personal view. Br Med J 1988; 296: 1191.

26. Myers GS : Quoted by Zola IK, see ref. 29.

27. Howard : Quoted by Mould RF in Medical Anecdotes, Bristol, 1983, p. 105.

28. Carlyon WH : Disease prevention / health promotion - bridging the gap to wellness. Health Values 1984; 8: 27-30.

29. Zola IK : Medicine as an institution of social control. In: A Sociology of Medical Practice. Cox C, Mead A, Eds. Collier-Macmillan, London, 1975, pp. 170-185.

30. Cochrane A L, Holland W W: Validation of Screening Procedures Brit Med Bull 1971; 27: 3-8

CHAPTER 5

1. Skrabanek P : Demarcation of the absurd. Lancet 1986; i: 960-961.
2. Stalker D, Glymour C, Eds: Examining Holistic Medicine. Prometheus Books, Buffalo, New York, 1985.
3. Hsu FLK : Exorcising the Trouble Makers. Magic, Science and Culture. Greenwood Press, Westport, Connecticut, 1983.
4. Anon : Quackery: a $10 billion scandal. A report by the chairman of the subcommittee of health and long-term care of the select committee of aging of the House of Representatives. 98th Congress, 2nd session. Publ. no. 98-435. U.S. Government Printing Office, Washington, 1984.
5. Braun A : Capsicum, das Heimweh und die Purifikatoren. Z klass Homöopath 1983; 27: 195-200.
6. Boyd H : Homoeopathic medicine. In: Alternative Therapies. Lewith G T, Ed. Heinemann, London, 1985, pp. 150-177.
7. von Baeyer HC : Caesar's last breath. Sciences, Vol 26, 1986, No. 6, pp. 2-4.
8. Anon : Homoeopathy gone mad. Med. Press 1879; 78: 256.
9. Vithoulkas G : Homoeopathy: a theory for the future? World Health Forum 1983; 4: 99-101.
10. Holmes DW : Homoeopathy. In: Examining Holistic Medicine. Stalker D and Glymour C, Eds. Prometheus Books, Buffalo, New York, 1985, pp. 221-242.

11. Simpson JY : Homoeopathy: Its Tenets and Tendencies. 3rd Edn. Sutherland and Knox, Edinburgh, 1853.

12. Anon : Homoeopathy and homoeopathic writings. Dublin Quart J Med Sci 1846; 1: 173-210.

13. Davenas E, et al. : Human basophil degranulation triggered by very dilute antiserum against IgE. Nature 1988; 333: 816-818.

14. Maddox J, Randi J, Stewart WW : 'High-dilution' experiments a delusion. Nature 1988; 334: 287-290.

15. Dorizynski A : French scientists say little; the French press, too much. Scientist, Sept 5th, 1988, p.4.

16. Reilly DT : Explanation of Benveniste. Nature 1988; 334: 285.

17. Vlamis G : Flowers to the Rescue. The Healing Vision of Dr Edward Bach. Thorsons, Wellingborough, 1986.

18. Skrabanek P : Acupuncture: past, present and future. In: Examining Holistic Medicine. Stalker D and Glymour G, Eds. Prometheus Books, Buffalo, New York, 1985.

19. Qian W-Y : The Great Inertia; Scientific Stagnation in Traditional China. Croom Helm, London, 1985.

20. Ackerknecht EH : Zur Geschichte der Akupunktur. Anaesthetist 1974; 23: 37-38.

21. Anon : Endorphins through the eye of a needle? Editorial. Lancet 1981; i: 480-482.

22. Skrabanek P : Acupuncture and endorphins. Lancet 1984; i: 220.

23. Skrabanek P : Acupuncture and the age of unreason. Lancet 1984; i: 1169-1171.

24. Skrabanek P : L'acupuncture. Journal International de Médicine. 1985; 10: 99.

25. Skrabanek P : Acupuncture - needless needles. Editorial. Irish Med J 1986; 79: 334-335.

26. Vora D : Health in your Hands. Acupressure Therapy (reflexol - ogy). 3rd Edn. Gala Publishers, Bombay, 1984.

27. Lewith GT : Acupuncture and other new diagnostic systems. Irish Medical Times, Jan 30, 1987, p 18.

28. Barker AT : Medical devices and consumer protection. Lancet 1987; i: 452.

29. Palmer DD : Textbook of the Science, Art and Philosophy of Chiropractic for Students and Practitioners. Portland Printing House Co., Portland, 1910.

30. Biemiller AJ : Fact sheet on chiropractic. JAMA 1970; 214: 1095-1096.

31. Mencken HL : Chiropractic. In: Prejudices, 6th Series. Cape, London, 1928, pp. 217-227.

32. Barrett S : Chiropractic. New Engl J Med 1976; 294: 346.

33. Gibson T, Grahame R, Harkness J, Woo P, Blagrave P and Hills R: Controlled comparison of short-wave diathermy with osteopathic treatment in non-specific low back pain. Lancet 1985; i: 1258-1261.

34. Bloch M : The Royal Touch. Sacred Monarchy and Scrofula in England and France. Translated by J.E.Andersen. Routledge & Kegan Paul, London, 1973.

35. Aubrey J : Miscellanea. 2nd Edn. Bettesworth and Battley, London, 1721.

36. Thorndike L : A History of Magic and Experimental Science, Vol 1, Macmillan, London, 1923.

37. Idem. Vol 7 Columbia Univ. Press, New York 1958.

38. Idem. Vol 8 Columbia Univ. Press, New York 1958.

39. Anon : Exploring the effectiveness of healing.
Lancet 1985; ii: 1177-1178.

40. Forbes A : Cymatics. In: A Visual Encyclopaedia of Unconventional Medicine. Hill A, Ed. New English Library, London,1979, p.180.

41. Charles, HRH Prince : Drugs - the patient has had enough. The Times, Dec 16, 1982, p. 12.

42. Bloom M : Oral Roberts' medical centre: merging medicine and prayer. Med World News, Dec 21, 1981, pp. 53-63.

43. Gardner R : Miracles of healing in Anglo-Celtic Northumbria as recorded by the Venerable Bede and his contemporaries: a reappraisal in the light of 20th century experience.
Br Med J 1983; 287: 1927-1933.

44. Brandon R : The Spiritualists. Weidenfield and Nicolson, London, 1983, p. 222.

45. Galton F : Statistical inquiries into the efficacy of prayer.
Fortnightly Review, Vol 12, No 68 (new series), August 1   1872, pp.125-135.

46. Joyce CRB, Welldon RMC : The objective efficacy of prayer.
     J Chron Dis 1965; 18: 367-377.

47. Talbot NA : The position of the Christian Science Church. New
     Engl J Med 1983; 309: 1641-1644.

48. Eddy MB : Science and Health with Key to the Scriptures. 89th
     Edn. The First Church of Christ Scientist, Boston, 1971.

49. Currier RD : Christian Science and the care of children.
     New Engl J Med 1984; 310: 1258.

50. Wilson GE : Christian Science and longevity.
     J Forensic Sci 1956; 1: 43-60.

51. Rose L : Faith Healing. Penguin Books, Harmondsworth, 1971.

52. Twain M : Christian Science (1907), in: The works of Mark Twain
     Vol 19. Baender P, Ed.
     University of California Press, Los Angeles, 1973.

53. Meek GW : Healers and the Healing Process. The Theosophical
     Publishing House, Wheaton, Illinois, 1977.

54. Watson L : Is primitive medicine really primitive? In: The
     Frontiers of Science and Medicine. Carlson RJ, Ed.
     Wildwood House, London, 1975.

55. Hill A, Ed: A Visual Encyclopaedia of Unconventional Medicine,
     New English Library, London, 1979.

56. Lloyd GER : Magic, Reason and Experience. Studies in the Origin
     and Development of Greek Science. Cambridge Univ. Press,
     Cambridge, 1979.

57. Nolen WA : Psychic Surgery. In: Science and Paranormal. Abell GO, Singer B, Eds. New York, 1981, pp. 185-1955.

58. Randi J : Flim-Flam: Psychics, Unicorns, and Other Delusions. Prometheus Books, Buffalo, New York, 1982.

59. Tansley DV : Dimension of Radionics : Health Science Press, Bradford, 1977.

60. Tomlinson H : Medical Divination. Theory and Practice. Health Science Press, Rustington, 1966.

61. Mason K : Radionics and Progressive Energies. Daniel, Saffron Walden, England, 1984.

62. Reyner JH : Psionic Medicine. The study and Treatment of the Causative Factors in Illness. 2nd Edn. Routledge and Kegan Paul, London, 1982.

63. Garrett A : The paranormal: fact or fantasy? The Skeptic 1986; 6 no.4: 18-20.

CHAPTER 6

1. Wolpert L : Science and anti-science, The Lloyd-Roberts Lecture 1986. J Roy Coll Physicians London 1987; 21: 159-165.

2. Ortega y Gasset J : The Mission of the University. Kegan Paul, London, 1946.

3. Black D : An Anthology of False Antitheses. Rock Carling Monograph. Nuffield Provincial Hospitals Trust, London, 1984.

4. Mencken HL : Prejudices. Third series. Jonathan Cape, London, 1923.

5. Foucault M : The Birth of the Clinic. Tavistock Publications, London, 1973.

6. Tissot : Quoted by Foucault, see 5.

7. Christen AG, Swanson BZ, Glover ED, Henderson AH : Smokeless tobacco: the folklore and social history of snuffing, sneezing, dipping, and chewing. J Am Dental Assoc 1982; 105: 821-825.

8. Picker H : The Hitler Phenomenon. David and Charles, Newton Abbot, 1974.

CHAPTER 7

1.   Bierce A : The cynic's Word Book. Doubleday, Page and
     Co., London, 1906.

2.   Dollery C : The End of an Age of Optimism. Rock Carling
     Monograph. Nuffield Provincial Hospitals Trust, London, 1978.

3.   The past and present of the medical profession.
     Boston Med Surg J 1851; 44: 338.

4.   Hobbes T : Leviathan, 1651.

QUOTATION ACKNOWLEDGEMENTS

Grateful acknowledgement is made to the following for permission to reproduce material in this book:

Annals of Internal Medicine (Chapter 2 Reference 36)
Mrs Margaret Asher (Chapter 1 Reference 5)
Blackwell Scientific Publications, Inc. (Chapter 1 Reference 17)
The British Medical Journal (Chapter 2 Reference 49)
Professor W W Holland (Chapter 4 Reference 30)
The Lancet (Chapter 2 Reference 23; Chapter 3 Reference 32)
The New England Journal of Medicine (Chapter 2 Reference 48; Chapter 3 Reference 12; Chapter 5 Reference 49)
Science (Chapter 3 Reference 20 - Copyright 1985 by the AAAS)
The Sunday Times (Chapter 4 Reference 7)